P9-BZJ-211

OCT   1995

BRAINSCAPES

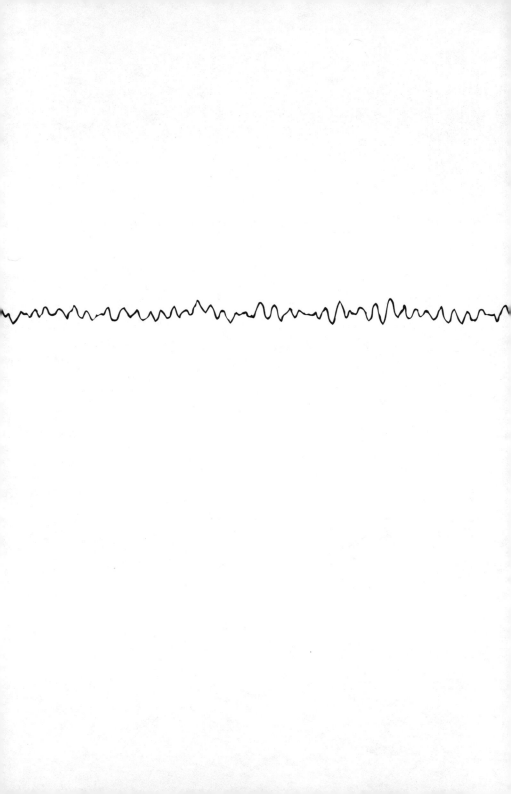

BRAINSCAPES

An Introduction to What
Neuroscience Has Learned
about the Structure, Function,
and Abilities of the Brain

RICHARD M. RESTAK, M.D.

A **Discover** BOOK

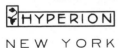HYPERION

NEW YORK

Brainscapes is the first in a series of books to be published by Hyperion in conjunction with *Discover* magazine, concerning the central issues of modern science.

Library of Congress Cataloging–in–Publication Data
Restak, Richard M.
Brainscapes : an introduction to what neuroscience has learned about the structure, function, and abilities of the brain / Richard M. Restak.—1st ed.
p.   cm.
Includes index.
ISBN 0-7868-6113-4
1. Brain—Popular works. 2. Intellect—Popular works. I. Title.
QP376.R4725 1995
612.8'2—dc20
95-14774
CIP

BOOK DESIGN BY BRIAN MULLIGAN

First Edition

10 9 8 7 6 5 4 3 2 1

To my mother, Alice Hynes Restak,
with love and gratitude

BRAINSCAPES

I

The Socratic maxim "know thyself," when translated into contemporary terms, demands that we know about our brain, thus converting a scientific discipline, neuroscience (the study of the brain), into a humanistic one. Such an enterprise was impossible until recently because we had very little knowledge of the brain. What knowledge we did have seemed unrelated to everyday concerns. But in the past twenty years scientists have learned more about the brain than they have in the previous two hundred; moreover, they have discovered that such familiar processes as thought, emotion, memory, perception, and all other expressions of mind cannot take place without reference to the brain.

Thus, an understanding of our brain and its organization can change us from being a passive member of the audience to that of the director who functions as an active observer of all of the things occurring both on and off the stage.

First, a fundamental principle: The brain exists in order to provide an internal representation of "reality." Quotation marks are employed here in deference to the fact that no creature, including ourselves, can ever know any other "reality" than the representations made by his brain. These representations, in turn, depend upon the brain's organization, which differs from one creature to another and, in our own species, from one person to another.

A second fundamental principle: Certain recurring themes have dominated the theories of those who have studied the brain and its importance in achieving self-understanding. Throughout history different ideas have been favored concerning the significance of the brain in the conduct of everyday life.

The Egyptians believed the heart and not the brain recorded all good and evil deeds. At the moment of death the heart was placed on a scale and weighed against a feather. The heart would be found to be either heavy with evil or, if free from evil deeds, as light as the feather. The brain was held in such disrepute that it was siphoned out through the nose of cadavers by means of a crude suction apparatus.

Not until the fifth century B.C. was the importance of the brain recognized by physicians like Alcmaeon and philosophers like Anaxagoras. In his *On the Sacred Disease* Hippocrates firmly equated the brain with the mind:

> Men ought to know that from nothing else but the brain comes joys, delights, laughter and sports, and sorrows, griefs, despondency, and lamentations. And by this, in an especial manner, we acquire wisdom and knowledge, and see and hear and know what are foul and what are fair, what are bad and what are good, what are sweet, and what are unsavory. . . . And by the same organ we become mad and delirious, and fears and terrors assail us. . . . All these things we endure from the brain, when it is not healthy. . . . In these ways I am of the opinion that the brain exercises the greatest power in the man.

This is the interpreter to us of those things which emanate from the air, when the brain happens to be in a sound state.

Plato took a different approach and postulated the existence of a triune soul. One part, associated with the intellect, resided in the brain; the second part, associated with fear, pride, anger, and courage, resided in the liver; the third part, related to lust, greed, and intemperate desire, dwelled even lower down in the intestine. While the soul of the liver and the soul of the gut perished at death, the intellectual, or rational, soul located in the brain was immortal.

Aristotle, Plato's pupil, differed from his teacher and resurrected the minority view favoring the heart as the seat of the soul or mind. The heart felt warm to the touch, the brain cold, Aristotle observed. And since warmth was associated in the Greek mind with sensation, the heart was annointed as the seat of the mind. Aristotle's influence survives today through metaphor. I am writing these words three days before Valentine's Day. No doubt I would have great difficulty finding a card depicting Cupid piercing a brain with his love arrows.

Galen, the physician to the Roman gladiators, favored the brain as the crucial organ in humans for practical reasons: He encountered firsthand the brain damage resulting from head wounds. He also carried out his own experiments. Since the performance of autopsies (a word Galen coined) was forbidden by Roman law, he substituted brain dissections on Barbary apes (chosen because, when walking or running, the creatures resembled humans more than any other primates known at the time).

Galen noted the similarities in the cerebral convolutions in man and ape but allowed himself to get sidetracked in a comical dispute about the relationship of brain convolutions to intelligence. Since donkeys possess complex cerebrums and they are exceedingly stupid animals, Galen decided that nothing could be concluded about intelligence from studying brain convolutions. Two thousand years later phrenologists who speculated about the brain on the basis of skull configurations would take the opposing argument to an extreme: they held the mistaken notion that not only intelligence but such specific traits as "destructiveness," "acquisitiveness," and "veneration" could be reliably gauged by palpating a person's skull and thereby divining the size and configuration of the underlying brain areas.

Today we know that Galen and the phrenologists were not entirely wrong in their belief that certain parts of the brain are specialized. Thanks to the discoveries of Paul Broca and Carl Wernicke, two nineteenth-century neuroanatomists, we have learned that the left cerebral hemisphere is important in language. Like Galen these two early brain researchers based their work on the examination of injured brains. They studied at autopsy the brains of patients who during their lives had suffered from language disorders. The left frontal and temporal areas, named after Broca and Wernicke respectively, are responsible for the production and comprehension of speech.

Throughout the nineteenth century neuroscientists argued whether the brain operates as a whole (i.e., organized holistically) or whether it can be partitioned like a map of Europe into separate domains, each having a specific function. As a measure of the difficulty of determining which theory was true, consider what you might conclude about a person who, after brain damage, lost the ability to recognize any numbers higher than three. (This is a real example that stimulated controversy at the turn of the century.) If you are a strict believer in localization, you might believe that only the parts of the brain containing memory images for the numbers one, two, and three remained undamaged while areas associated with all other numbers had been destroyed.

A more holistic interpretation was favored by a neurologist, Jacques Loeb, who reasoned that the numbers one, two, and three had a series of associations that extended throughout the cerebrum and thus were more resistant to injury of a single part of the brain. He wrote: "In processes of association the cerebral hemispheres act as a whole, and not as a mosaic of a number of different parts. . . . Association processes occur everywhere in the hemispheres."

After much debate the supporters of localization temporarily refuted the arguments set forth by Loeb and others, at least in regard to sensations, movement, and language. Other areas were subsequently linked with *vision* (the occipital lobe and surrounding association fibers); *hearing* (the temporal lobes); *touch, bodily sensation,* and the formation of a *body image* (the parietal lobes); *facial recognition* (the right parietal lobe); and other faculties.

Such discoveries did not come quickly nor were they readily accepted. But as we shall see, controversy still persists today regarding the origin of behavior, consciousness, and an integrated sense of self. None of these more abstract qualities has ever been strictly localized, although they are dependent for their full expression on the normal functioning of certain brain areas.

The holism-localization dichotomy represents a dialectic in the sense that Hegel used that term: a continuing dynamic opposition of opposites. Thus both theories about the brain are correct in their own way: the brain is specialized and yet at the same time operates as a whole.

Over the centuries our ancestors studied the intact brain in its natural state. With the invention of the microscope its smaller and finer details could be observed. Accompanying the experiments and observations came sometimes fanciful speculations about the interrelationships of brain, mind, and soul. This was a natural consequence of the brain's inaccessibility. It sits within the bony vault of our cranium, the skull, surrounded by three membrane layers, the *meninges.*

The outermost layer, the *dura mater* (Latin for "hard mother"), is a tough covering with the consistency of leather that anchors the brain to the inside of the skull. It also contains many blood vessels that shear in response to head injuries. The clotted blood that accumulates between the dura and brain (a condition called *subdural hematoma)* leads to paralysis, coma, and finally death if it is not removed. Prior to the advent of neurosurgery only little more than

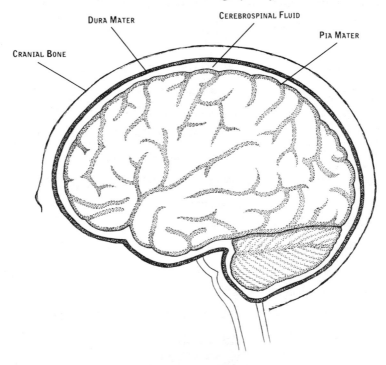

DURA MATER   CEREBROSPINAL FLUID

PIA MATER

CRANIAL BONE

125 years ago, that removal was done crudely and hastily by drilling a hole through the bone. This process, called *trephination,* allowed the clot to escape outward rather than tunnel inward.

The innermost layer, the *pia mater* (Latin for "tender mother"), is a thin delicate membrane that inspired some early neuroanatomist with a poetical bent to compare the way this membrane envelops the brain to the gentleness of a mother caressing her infant. Shakespeare was familiar with this most intimate of the brain's components. In *Love's Labour's Lost* Holofernes says:

"This is a gift that I have, simple, simple; a foolish extravagant spirit, full of forms, figures, shapes, objects, ideas, apprehensions, motions, revolutions; these are begot in the ventricle of memory, nourished in the womb of pia mater, and delivered upon the mellowing of occasion."

Between the outer dura mater and the inner pia mater lies a reticulated layer of tissue, *the arachnoid,* whose appearance reminded another now-anonymous anatomist of a spider's web. Between this arachnoid layer and the pia mater flows a river of cerebrospinal fluid that bathes the brain and provides a soft, fluid, protective cushion. The cerebrospinal fluid originates from the walls of an interconnected cave located deep within the brain. The chambers of this cave, the *ventricles,* are four in number: each of the two lateral ventricles is located at the lowermost point of one of the two cerebral hemispheres, while the third ventricle is a midline slit that extends downward into the brain stem to communicate with the fourth ventricle.

Scholastics and mystics in the Middle Ages conjectured about the purpose of the ventricles and their place in the operation of the mind. They considered that thought, an immaterial substance, must originate immaterially, and thus believed the "empty" ventricles (they were unaware of the cerebrospinal fluid) served as the originator and conduit of thought. In a materialistic age such as ours a theory based on "emptiness" over one founded on substance may seem anomalous and even bizarre. I have in my collection of prints and lithographs about the brain one image that makes such reasoning more understandable if not necessarily more acceptable. It shows God in the heavens thinking the Word, as St. John employed the term (i.e., all of reality), and a transmission of this message from Heaven to humankind, where it enters the brain via the hollow ventricles wherein dwelled the equally incorporeal human mind.

A variation on this theory of the brain and nervous system, favored by Galen, involved a series of pneumatic tubes that conducted animal spirits from the ventricles to various parts of the body. Digested food, after transfer from the gut to the liver, was transformed into natural spirits. The natural spirits then passed to the right side of the heart for conversion to vital spirits. After passage to the brain's ventricles via the arteries, vital spirits were converted into animal spirits, which passed along the hollow nerves to force muscles into action or convey sensation.

While such a theory about the brain seems incredibly fantastic today, it dominated thought, at least in the West, for over fifteen hundred years. It could do so only because it appeared to explain certain observations. For instance, the observation that brain activity ceased coincident with a blockage of blood supply to the organ was taken as proof that the vital spirits could no longer wend their way to the brain from the rest of the body.

Belief in an invisible "spirit" continued in a modified form and captured the imagination of students of the brain during the eighteenth and nineteenth centuries. In 1678 Jan Schwammerdam showed the Grand Duke of Tuscany that a frog's leg muscle contracted when it and its nerve were mounted on a copper support and touched to the support by means of wires twisted around the muscle. Later, Luigi Galvani extended these observations in an experiment that today sounds like something out of a low-budget horror movie.

In November 1780, Galvani erected a long, insulated iron wire antenna on the roof of his house. Dead frogs were connected both to the antenna and to another wire that led to the water in a nearby well. When lightning flashed in the sky, electricity traveled along the conductor and several frogs' muscles contracted. Later Galvani simplified his experiments even more: frogs hung by bronze hooks that penetrated their spinal cords went into contractions when placed on iron gratings. He suggested "animal electricity" (reminiscent of "animal spirits") as the force responsible for conduction along the nerve and the resultant stimulation of the muscle.

The invention of the galvanometer made possible the measurement of small current flows secondary to differences in potential (voltage) between two terminals. Disappointingly, no current flow could be detected in living tissue, but it was only because the instruments lacked the necessary sensitivity; not until 1840 was the galvanometer refined enough to prove that tiny currents did flow in the nerves.

Contemporaneous with these discoveries about the physiology— i.e., function—of the brain were declarations made by eighteenth-century phrenologists, who held forth on all of the marvelous insights made possible by taking external measurements of the shape of the skull. A nineteenth-century lithograph in my possession shows a post-dinner-party entertainment in Edinburgh, Scotland, during which the participants palpate one another's skulls and compare their findings with established charts purporting to reveal the meanings of each skull's configuration. Today we snicker at such naïveté, but explorers of the brain one hundred years from now are just as likely to find our divisions equally arbitrary and nonsensical. For our current understanding of the brain we rely on cartography, geography, and what can be seen with the naked eye and sketched with the hand. Later we will discuss why true knowledge may require reliance on a clever understanding of the brain's process—the millisecond communication within the networks of nerve cells widespread throughout the brain. Nonetheless, some plan of organization must be agreed upon in the interest of providing the basis for a clear overview, and the following offers a useful Baedeker's to the brain's geography:

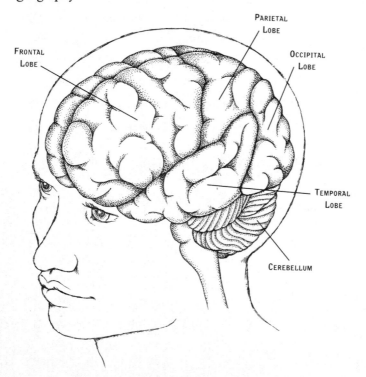

Viewed from the side, each of the overarching cerebral hemispheres of the brain resembles an old, wrinkled boxing glove. The front, middle, and back of the glove correspond to the brain's frontal, parietal (from the Latin for "wall"), and occipital ("back of the head") lobes, while the thumb of the boxing glove corresponds to the temporal lobe.

The *frontal* lobe makes up 50 percent of the volume of each cerebral hemisphere in humans. It initiates all motor activity, including speech; its most anterior divisions, the prefrontal lobes and supplementary motor cortex, integrate personality with emotion and transform thought into action.

Each *parietal* lobe is the receiving station for sensory information from the opposite side of the body and is responsible for the integration of what is seen with what is felt via a network of association fibers.

The *temporal* lobe is concerned with hearing and merges with structures such as the entorhinal cortex, the amygdala, and the hippocampus, which are involved in learning, memory and the experience and expression of emotion.

Finally, the *occipital* lobe, farthest to the back of the brain, processes visual perception.

Viewed from the top, the brain resembles a piece of sea coral, split down the middle by a great division, the longitudinal fissure. By means of this "Grand Canyon" the cerebrum is more or less divided into two cerebral hemispheres subdivided on each side into its four lobes comprising the *cerebral cortex;* the *basal ganglia;* and the *diencephalon.* While we share the latter two structures with other species (traditionally but inaccurately described as "lower" than ourselves; inaccurate because the brain of each creature is marvelously adapted to the environment in which it finds itself), the cerebral cortex is rudimentary in every creature other than humans.

A gray cellular mantle less than five millimeters in thickness, the cortex is the part of the brain containing the "little gray cells" to which Agatha Christie's detective Hercule Poirot was fond of referring, the neurons that make us who we are and make possible our poetry and philosophy, along with all of the madcap schemes for self- and species preservation and advancement ever hatched by Homo sapiens.

If the parts of the human body are sketched onto the brain surface corresponding to the amount of tissue that serves each part, a bizarre and distorted caricature is produced. The neurosurgeon Wilder Penfield, who carried out the operating-room experiments demonstrating how the brain is partitioned according to function, referred to the distorted figure as an homunculus. The strangeness of the figure stems from the fact that the motor and sensory areas of the hemispheres are

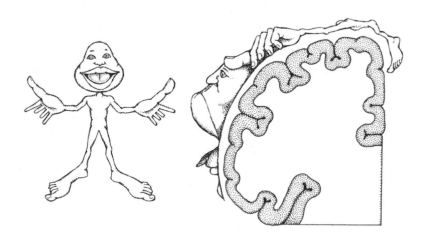

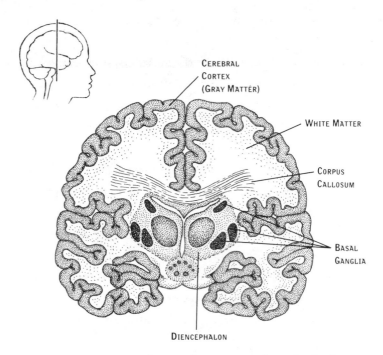

CEREBRAL
CORTEX
(GRAY MATTER)

WHITE MATTER

CORPUS
CALLOSUM

BASAL
GANGLIA

DIENCEPHALON

organized so as to emphasize those parts of our body that are most important to us. Since we are verbal creatures, large motor and sensory areas are dedicated to the lips, tongue, and pharynx. Similarly, because of our ability to manipulate tools and perform feats of fine hand and finger coordination, extensive cerebral areas are devoted to sensation and movement involving our four fingers and thumb.

A significant area of brain research has attempted to answer the fundamental question: But which came first? Is our brain organized as a reflection of our species' special talents, or are our abilities the result of our brain's organization? Resolving this conundrum is a little like deciding which came first, the chicken or the egg. Our brain's organization both reflects our species' existence on this planet while at the same time determining for us the nature of our "reality."

Beneath the hemispheres lie the basal ganglia, clusters of neurons huddled together into structures with exotic Latin names like *cau-date, putamen, globus pallidus,* and *claustrum.*

They are most closely linked with the initiation, smoothness, and precision of movement, and are responsible for the automatic movements we make without thinking. Turning the pages of this book, withdrawing from the sting of a scorpion, dancing to the rhythm of a familiar song while thinking of events that occurred earlier in the day—it's the basal ganglia that make such responses possible. Disturbances here are responsible for the tremor, slowness, and general difficulty of "getting started" characteristic of Parkinson's disease.

If, however, we decide to focus attention on the act of page turning, to examine and classify the insect that bit us, or to dance to an *un*familiar tune, our basal ganglia must consult the cortex to make these more subtle and intellectual processes possible. In fact, the cerebrum and basal ganglia are engaged continuously in two-way interaction.

Connecting the two cerebral hemispheres is the *corpus callosum,* a large rope of nerve fibers conveying information in both directions. The corpus callosum takes over a decade to fully mature, thus limiting information transfer in a young child's brain. This delayed maturation is one explanation for why few of us have memories that go back into infancy or very early childhood. It also accounts for why very young children perform poorly on tests in which they must transfer information from one hemisphere to another, such as pointing with the right hand to objects felt with the left hand. Later we will take up in more detail the intriguing findings and theories resulting from severing the corpus callosum.

Located below the back part of the cerebrum is the *cerebellum,* sometimes called the "little brain," the area most concerned with balance, posture, and the coordination of movement. It consists of a large mass of closely packed folia (leaflike bundles of nerve cells) divided into two hemispheres joined by a finger-shaped structure called the *vermis*. As with the cerebral hemispheres, nerve impulses from the cerebellum follow a crossed pathway, (i.e., from the right cerebellar hemisphere to the left cerebral hemisphere, from the left cerebellar hemisphere to the right cerebral hemisphere).

A starlike structure, the brain stem, connects the cerebrum with the spinal cord. At its upper end are the *thalamus* and *hypothalamus*, once poetically compared to the inner or bridal chamber of the house, and the room immediately beneath it. Both thalamus and hypothalamus are components of the limbic system, a group of inter-connected regions in the cortex and the area below it responsible for some aspects of memory and the experience and expression of emo-tion. There are actually two thalami, one on each side of the brain. Both receive all sensory impulses except smell from one side of the body and route them to the appropriate areas of the cerebral cortex.

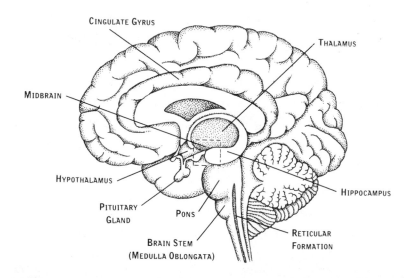

The thalami also relay impulses from one part of the brain to another in a feedback arrangement.

The hypothalamus is much smaller, no more than one three-hundredth of the total brain, but despite its diminutive size it is responsible for regulating such critical functions as body temperature, hunger, sexuality, and, via connections with the nearby pituitary gland (the "master gland of the body"), the endocrine system and the composition of the blood and fluid compartments, that internal symphony of circulating chemicals in our bodies aptly described by the French physiologist Claude Bernard as the "internal milieu."

Just below the thalamus and hypothalamus is the midbrain, which controls movement of the eyes and the size of the pupils. Further down is the pons, so named because of its fancied resemblance to a bridge spanning a river. Observed from the front it reaches from one side of the brain stem to the other, the ends disappearing into the mass of tissue toward the cerebellum. It contains ascending and descending fibers linking the cerebrum with the rest of the brain. The bottom part of the brain stem, merging with the spinal cord, is the *medulla oblongata*. Within this inch of nervous system lie the centers for breathing, heart rate, vomiting, and the articulation of speech and song. It is here that the major pathways for sensation and movement cross over, ensuring for some so-far-inexplicable reason that each cerebral hemisphere controls the opposite side of the body.

Deep within the brain stem and ascending upward is a complex and loosely arranged collection of cells, the reticular formation, that regulates the brain's level of awareness. Sensory impulses that pass along the brain stem stimulate the reticular formation, which in turn activates the brain and maintains wakefulness and alertness.

From the brain stem emerge ten of the twelve cranial nerves, excluding the optic and olfactory (the nerves governing sight and smell, deliver information directly from the nose and eyes for pro-cessing by the brain). These ten nerves spread to the head, neck, and torso where they move the eyes, and provide conduits for facial sen-sation and movement, hearing, swallowing, and the activation of glands and muscles.

Of course we are not entirely (or even, some would claim, pre-dominantly) intellectual creatures. We feel as well as cogitate. To locate the brain areas that control emotion, imagine the brain cut down the middle, through the "Grand Canyon," and then one half laid out before you like a grapefruit set out on your breakfast plate.

The *limbic system*, the mediator of all things emotional, consists of interconnected cortical and subcortical regions at the center of the brain. Think of a poet's sensitivity to nuance combined with the visu-ally imaginative skills of the architect and the cartographer if you wish to understand the contribution of the limbic system. Neuroscientists, lacking one or more of these skills, still argue at international meet-ings about whether they have identified *all* of the structures com-prising the limbic system. No one even suspected its existence until 1715, when the Dutch physician and chemist Herman Boerhaave noted that patients who had been bitten by rabid animals began "gnashing their teeth and snarling like a dog." At autopsy the brains of such unfortunates, as well as those of animals with rabies, were markedly inflamed in portions of the limbic system. Boerhaave's observations were not clarified until two centuries later when a French neurologist, Henri Gastaut, showed that rabies, then known to be caused by a virus, infects regions of the limbic system.

In 1937 a more scientific exposition was provided by anatomist James Papez. In a mellifluous burst of phrasing unusual for a brain expert he enthused that the hypothalamus, the anterior thalamic nucleus, the cingulate gyrus, the hippocampus, and their interconnections constitute "a harmonious mechanism which may elaborate the functions of central emotions as well as participate in emotional expressions." Neuroanatomist Paul MacLean expanded this definition of the limbic system to include the structures shown in the illustration on page 15.

(As an indication of the relative youth of neuroscience, MacLean, at eighty-two years of age, is still conducting brain research. Nor is he unique in this regard, since over 90 percent of all of the brain scientists who have ever lived are still living today. Moreover, more has been learned about the brain in the past twenty years than in the previous two hundred. How humbling, as well as exciting, to realize that one of the greatest insights into our internal organization—the discovery of the limbic system—dates back only slightly more than half a century.)

In practical terms the most important limbic regions are associated with the temporal lobe: the hippocampus, amygdala, and areas in the immediate surroundings. Fibers from all four lobes, along with association fibers uniting these separate connections into one unified experience, converge into the hippocampal region. Within that structure multiple connections are formed and feedback fibers are projected to the lobes and association fibers, as well as to other limbic structures where emotions are forged.

Thanks to extensive two-way connections, with other brain areas the hippocampus and its immediate connecting structures integrate and coordinate both our outer- and inner-world experiences into a unity. Damage to the hippocampus on both sides of the brain deprives the victim of the ability to learn new things and thus suspends the person in a time warp composed of the distant past, a present as thin and sharply etched as a knife blade, and an uncertain and fearful future. This happens because under normal circumstances we are able to maintain our sense of identity—who we *are*—only by forming new memories from moment to moment and accessing old ones at a leisurely command. It is precisely the loss of identity, secondary to a devastated memory, that occasions such sadness and dismay in the relatives of the Alzheimer's victim; they recognize that the person whom they knew and loved, but who no longer recognizes them, has ceased to exist.

It has always seemed appropriate to me that the psychic depths of our emotional experiences should be mirrored by the brain's organization: the areas responsible for feelings found deepest, darkest, and most central, with our more rational thoughts and mental processes emanating from our cerebral hemispheres, particularly the cerebral cortices. Thus in this analogy we "ascend" from the influence of our emotions located in the interior limbic structures up toward the "higher" brain centers. But such metaphorical thinking shouldn't be taken too far. Thoughts and emotions are interwoven: every thought, however bland, almost always carries with it some emotional undertone, however subtle.

In the 1890s John Hughlings Jackson, a neurologist with philosophical training (he studied with Herbert Spencer), suggested that the cerebral cortex held in check the more "primitive" impulses, such as sex and aggression, that originate in these underlying structures. Jackson spoke of the "release" of these older, deeper structures following damage to the cerebral cortex. This was a brilliant and prescient insight, since at the time Jackson had no certainty of the action of those areas that would later be understood to be part of the limbic system. Freud, who was also a neurologist, would later incorporate Jackson's "hierarchical" framework into his psychoanalytic theory. The ego, and more especially the superego, corresponded to the functioning of the cerebral cortex, while the "impulses" of the id smoldered in the depths of the brain, from whence they erupted during nightmares and psychotic episodes.

Although we know a lot about the brain in regard to the size and position of its various components, this tells us little about how the organ actually works. While we have discovered a great deal about its function, any theory can never be more than a best estimate at the time, since additional technological advances will make available new information and new ways of thinking about long-held knowledge. A summary of our present understanding of the brain's operations would go something like this:

If the brain is considered from the point of view of complexity, four different levels of functioning exist for the human cortex, the outer 3 to 5 millimeters of the cerebral hemispheres that play the major role in determining who we are and what we can do. Each of these four divisions has its own anatomical boundaries and distinctive principles of operation.

The *primary cortex* is the simplest zone and consists of islands of brain tissue that process sensory stimulation of a single type—vision, hearing, and touch. Vision is located farthest, toward the rear of the brain; hearing, in the temporal lobes; and touch and other skin-mediated sensations, from the sensory tract just behind the motor strip.

Next in the order of complexity are the association areas related to each of the primary sensory areas, the *uni*modal cortex. It is in this region that elaborate and detailed sensory processing of sight, sound, and touch are made possible. But nothing in the way of an overall synthesis occurs at this level, since the three sensations are kept separate. A synthesis integrating each sensory input with the others occurs only at the *third* level: the *hetero*modal association cortex. This is a rich matrix of nerve fibers that forms a network that unites into a whole the individual contributions of the senses into a unified perception.

To get some idea of the contributions of those three areas of the cortex, imagine yourself staring at an image from about three inches away and experiencing nothing more than an isolated color—say, red (processed by the primary cortex). You then step back a few inches farther and appreciate that red is the color of a dress (processed by the *uni*modal visual cortex); finally you step back still farther—at the same moment the projectionist turns on the projector and engulfs you in the sights and sounds of a garden party (*hetero*modal association cortex). At this point you have the synthesis of what the red color and the dress are all about. Missing from your mental landscape is the *meaning* of your perception of the garden party, and what attitude you are going to take toward it. This *fourth* and highest level of human cognition depends upon the *supra*modal association cortex where behavioral control is exerted over all of the brain functions of the lower levels. This is located mainly in the frontal and prefrontal parts of the brain.

In addition to these four functional zones mental life is also dependent upon the action of the brain areas beneath the cortex. Levels of alertness and "cortical tone," referred to by neurologist Frank Benson as "the development and maintenance of an optimal state for higher cortical operations," depends upon the integrity of a midline track of fibers known as the reticular activating system (RAS). Wakefulness, drowsiness, and sleep correspond to variations in the influence of the RAS on the cerebral cortex. Injury or destruction of fibers in this tract results in a permanent state of coma, and disorders such as narcolepsy—the tendency toward uncontrollable episodes of sleep, often in inappropriate circumstances—are associated with EEG abnormalities in this area. Many subcortical circuits are responsible for cortical tone and include contributions from the limbic system, which governs the full alertness and readiness to respond that accompanies fear or anxiety.

A boxer provides an example of the multiple and interactive processes going on within the brain. First he must be fully alert and responsive to the dangers and opportunities of his environment. (A knockout results from a disruption of the influence of the RAS on higher brain structures.) As he moves out to the center of the ring the fighter integrates information from all sensory inputs, particularly vision, in order to produce an appropriate and timely motor response. Thanks to practice and training the responses occur on an unconscious reflex level governed principally by the basal ganglia. Indeed, automatic and instantaneous responsiveness is what distinguishes the professional from the amateur.

As the fighter engages with his opponent he relies upon the smooth functioning of multiple functional circuits integrated into networks. While most of these involve stimulation, others, no less important, mediate inhibition. (The fighter must ignore the cheers and jeers of the crowd and focus his full attention on his opponent.) Sensation is not separable from the motor response: a punch may be "pulled" at the last split second and another launched with the opposite hand in response to the other fighter momentarily dropping his guard. At all times the fighter's brain is integrating many sensory inputs and motor outputs in parallel motion rather than in a series of motions, and each of its operations influences all the others. The sum total of all of this activity forms a seamless, perceptual whole.

Brain Development

By eighteen days after the union of the man's sperm and the woman's egg a layer of the embryonic disc, the ectoderm, thickens along the back of the layer to form a neural plate of cells that elongates and closes in on itself along the sides and top to form the neural tube (the precursor of the brain) and its distant outpost, the spinal cord. By the end of the first embryonic month the brain resembles the sort of animal balloon beloved by children. Three prominent swellings mark the forebrain, the midbrain, and the hindbrain.

All cells within the brain originate from the lining of the neural tube. They migrate outward to form the gray matter, composed of the nerve cells, and the white matter, made up of bundles of nerve fibers traveling throughout the brain between different regions of gray matter.

Midway through fetal life the tubelike brain has filled out into a globular shape with three distinguishable features:

* three curvatures or flexures: the cephalic, the pontine, and the cervical
* the enlargement of certain areas, such as the cerebrum and the cerebellum, out of proportion to all of the others
* the downward overgrowth of the cerebral hemispheres, which serves to obscure from direct sight the midbrain and the hindbrain.

STAGES IN PRENATAL BRAIN DEVELOPMENT

25 DAYS   35 DAYS   40 DAYS   50 DAYS   100 DAYS

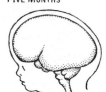 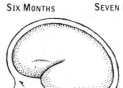 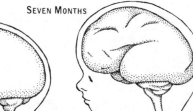

FIVE MONTHS   SIX MONTHS   SEVEN MONTHS

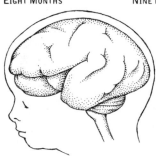 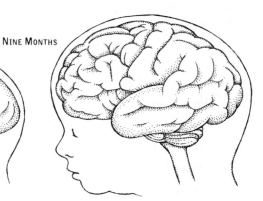

EIGHT MONTHS   NINE MONTHS

Next the cerebrum changes its appearance from something like the smooth ivory head of a walking stick to something resembling crumpled crepe paper. This alteration is dictated by the unlikely triumvirate of economics, obstetrics, and physics. More nerve cells can coexist in less space if surface area is increased without increasing volume. (The same principle of crumpling in order to contain large surface areas in a small volume is employed in the construction of parachutes.) In the brain the crumpling involves the outer cortical surface of the hemispheres into the fissures and the convolutions—gyri—that give the brain its gnarled-walnut appearance. By this means the brain can be kept small enough at birth to pass through the birth canal.

By the seventh month all the major demarcations are present and capable of being named, noted, and annotated. Indeed, by two years of age the size of the brain and its proportions are essentially the same as in an adult.

While the brain is often compared to a computer, no existing computer can do all of the things carried out by the brain. Consider just the stupendous complexity involved. How does one begin to comprehend the functioning of an organ with somewhere in the neighborhood of 50 billion neurons with a million billion synapses (connections), and with an overall firing rate of perhaps 10 million billion times per second? To put that in perspective, if those numbers hold true for the human mind, then a typical desktop computer is capable of the calculating power of a small snail, and the Cray 2, one of the fastest supercomputers in existence, possesses the processing power of a small rodent. The gulf is also vast between the brain and neural-network-based computers which, it is claimed, imitate the brain's organization of vast networks of nerve cells operating in parallel. The performance of even the most advanced of the neural-network computers is far inferior to that of the brain. The TRW Mark III, the most powerful of the neural-network computers built in the 1980s, and containing a million synapses, has about one ten-thousandth the mental capacity of a housefly.

No computer can match the operation of the brain because no computer can rewrite its own program; all computer forms of "thinking" are limited by the software operating at the time. The human brain, and the human brain alone, has the capacity to step back, survey its own operation, and thus achieve some degree of transcendence. Indeed, our capacity for rewriting our own script and redefining ourselves in the world is what distinguishes us from all other creatures in the world. It is our brain and its organization that makes that possible.

But what keeps our brain from being overwhelmed by all of the sensory information impinging upon it? Several self-protective reflexes exist. For one thing, and as we will discuss in detail later, information transfer within the brain occurs as a result of the passage of electrical impulses. A neuron, therefore, requires a certain amount of time for recovery between stimulations. During this "absolute refractory period," as it is called, a second nerve impulse cannot be generated. Furthermore, for a sensory stimulus to be perceived it must activate a critical mass of neurons joined together in circuits; it must also do so for a sufficient period of time.

A second factor preventing the brain from being overcome are certain "gating" mechanisms whereby inhibitory neurons modulate the influence of incoming sensory stimulation. Control of pain by means of acupuncture is one example of this mechanism with which neuroscientists are already familiar. Higher-level "gating" mechanisms have been proposed but not proven for narrowing the field of attention and concentration as in the boxer example mentioned above.

Competition for the same neurons and circuits provides a final safety valve, preventing the brain from being inundated by a deluge of sensory stimulation. This limits, for instance, the number of conversations that you can monitor when in a crowded room. And recall how much easier it is when you are on the telephone to have someone hand you a written note instead of standing before you and conveying the same information verbally—thus "jamming" the same circuits you're using during the phone conversation. Nor can any of us experience certain complementary emotions at the same time. It's not possible to be bored while excited, angry while serenely contented. We can certainly alternate rapidly from one to the other, but we cannot experience them *simultaneously*.

Competition involving circuits containing some of the same neurons also explains the incompatibility of certain emotions and thoughts. While thinking about the recent death or loss of someone we cared about we cannot experience happiness or elation; we may try to force "happy thoughts" about our loss but they remain just that: thoughts, and not internal emotional experiences.

At the highest level of thinking—conscious, directed attention— we can exclude outside sensory stimulation altogether. The writer intensely involved in the lives of her characters; the scuba diver who loses all sense of space and time while exploring the hulk of a sunken ship; the Grand Prix driver alert for that split second when he will make his move and overtake the leader: in each case external stimulation is narrowly focused and directed by internal, directed thought. But as everyone knows from experience the brain can only retain its intense focus for a certain period of time, a period that differs from one person to another. (One of the hallmarks of the peak performer is an ability to concentrate and focus longer than his opponent.)

As William James defined it, conscious, directed attention is "the taking possession by the mind, in clear and vivid form, of one out of what seem several simultaneously possible objects or trains of thought. Focalization, concentration, of consciousness are, of its essence." On most occasions and for most people this is a comparatively rare event. And, according to William James:

> The stream of our thought is like a river. On the whole easy simple flowing predominates in it, the drift of things is with the pull of gravity, and effortless attention is the rule. But at intervals an obstruction, a set-back, a log-jam occurs, stops the current, creates an eddy, and makes things temporarily move the other way. If a real river could feel, it would feel these eddies and set-backs as places of effort. "I am here flowing," it would say, "in the direction of greatest resistance, instead of flowing as usual in the direction of the least. My effort is what enables me to perform this feat."

While creative and successful people seem to have a greater capacity to focus their attention for prolonged periods of time, even the most humble of us can do so under conditions of threat or danger. (The prospect of an execution focuses the mind remarkably, suggested Samuel Johnson.) But such conditions are mercifully the exception during our normal waking mental life. Under most conditions, the mind's activities are similar to the description provided by J. M. Barrie of his attempts at a metaphor for a child's mind, an effort he undertook while preparing an adaptation of his play *Peter Pan:*

I don't know whether you have ever seen a map of a person's mind. Doctors sometimes draw maps of other parts of you, and your own map can become intensely interesting, but catch them trying to draw a map of a child's mind, which is not only confused, but keeps going round all the time. There are zigzag lines on it, just like your temperature on a card, and these are probably roads in the island; for the Neverland is always more or less an island, with astonishing splashes of color here and there, and coral reefs and rakish-looking craft in the offing, and savage and lonely lairs, and gnomes who are mostly tailors, and caves through which a river runs, and princes with six elder brothers, and a hut fast going to decay, and one very small old lady with a hooked nose. It would be an easy map if that were all; but there is also first day at school, religion, fathers, the round pond, needlework, murders, hangings, verbs that take the dative, chocolate pudding day, getting into braces, say ninety-nine, threepence for pulling out your tooth yourself, and so on; and either these are part of the island or they

are another map showing through, and it is all rather confus-
ing, especially as nothing will stand still.

Recent research employing positron emission tomography (PET)
scans, which provide color-coded pictures of ongoing brain activity,
reveals what is happening in the brain during times of concentrated
attention. (Such work is illustrative of the kinds of correlations
between our mental lives and brain functioning that neuroscientists
will be making in the future.) Imagine yourself sitting at a computer
console and staring at its screen. You have been instructed to press a
button the instant you detect a small cross on the screen. After some
practice at that you are given a cue (a brief flash) that indicates where
on the screen the cross is likely to appear next. Not only will your
responses to the cross now occur more quickly but measures of brain
electrical potential will be more robust. A PET scan will show
increased activation in the parietal lobe, a portion of the midbrain
(the superior colliculus), and the pulvinar, a nucleus in the thalamus.
    According to Michael Posner and Marcus Raichle, who have car-
ried out PET studies on attention, the parietal lobe releases attention from its current focus and signals the midbrain to move the
spotlight of attention toward the cued area. The pulvinar, a component of the basal ganglia, enhances and amplifies the attended target.
Together, these three components comprise the *posterior* attentional
network.
    An *anterior* attentional network is concerned with bringing the
object of attention into consciousness. (Obviously, we can be aware
of something but not necessarily consciously aware: we withdraw
our hand from the hot stove milliseconds before we either recognize
what we have done or felt the pain.) PET scan studies show that this
network consists of the anterior cingulate, located along the midline

of the frontal lobe; lateral parts of the frontal lobes; and parts of the basal ganglia. This anterior attention system is brought into play when only one of several competing decisions must be selected. (For this reason it is also called the executive network.) For instance, in an exercise called a Stroop Test, words for colors are written out in discongruent inks (i.e., "red" is printed in green ink), and the reader must name the color of ink while ignoring the printed word. (He must say "green" and thus ignore the printed "red.") To perform well in this test a person's anterior cingulate must come into play and inhibit the normal automatic tendency to read words and ignore ink colors. The more that we are consciously aware of what we are doing the more likely it is that the anterior attentional network is active. Posner and Raichle suggest in their book *Images of Mind* that "indeed it seems likely that the executive network is somehow related to our subjective experience of awareness. This sounds a great deal like what is meant by consciousness."

Consciousness in fact, is both readily accessible and mysterious. To experience it we have only to turn our attention inward, but in trying to explain it to others or prove its existence in persons other than ourselves, we immediately encounter a conundrum: language evolved for the most part to deal with aspects of the outer rather than the inner world.

When we attempt to describe the immediacy of our inner landscape we fall back on descriptions that mostly involve moment-to-moment reflections on what is happening around us, memories of the past, and anticipations of the future. Accompanying these are internal reflections that reveal various aspects of our character and emotional makeup. James Joyce in *Ulysses* and Virginia Woolf in *Mrs. Dalloway* perfected the "stream of consciousness" technique to portray states of mind. But neither Joyce nor Woolf "explained" consciousness; they merely presented what most of us accept as an accurate and prescient rendering of what we all experience during moments of inner awareness.

That word *awareness* is responsible, I believe, for much of our difficulty in coming to terms with consciousness. We often use these two terms as if they were the same thing; actually, they have quite different meanings. It is possible to be aware of something without being conscious of it. As we drive along a superhighway we are aware (or better be!) of all sorts of things about the flow of traffic around us. But unless we are a very inexperienced driver, or encounter something unexpected and potentially hazardous, we don't *consciously* attend to the other cars. For the most part we rely on routines and subroutines that we have learned over the years and buried deep in our basal ganglia to keep us *aware* but only intermittently *conscious* of the events surrounding our driving. Some deliberate mental effort as well as a certain period of time seem necessary for consciousness.

Experiments involving neurosurgical patients reveal that electrical impulses delivered to a part of the thalamus can be reliably detected by means of a forced choice ("Even if you're not sure, take a guess each time you sense the electrical stimulus") though the subject denies any conscious awareness of the stimulation. An additional duration of stimulation is required for a correct detection with awareness (a conscious response). In other words, the subject cannot simply choose, as in our driving example, to be conscious of the stimulation. Benjamin Libet, the neuroscientist who carried out the experiments, proposes that a certain duration or "time on" of neuronal activity may be one controlling factor separating conscious and unconscious functioning. Durations less than this minimum can result only in unconscious mental activity.

Conscious and unconscious mental processing also involve different parts of the brain: some brain areas seem more critical to consciousness than others. Localized brain damage can result in unexpected, even bizarre discrepancies between conscious and unconscious mental processing. For instance, an injury to the frontal medial cortex leads to a condition called the "alien hand syndrome," in which the injured person reaches out with a hand and grasps at something, or performs some other deliberate movement that is not consciously willed, and in most instances takes place autonomously and in defiance of the person's expressed wishes (hence the term *alien*). A fundamental principle emerges from cases like these, a principle that concerns not only consciousness but more generalized brain functioning as well. I'm referring to the distinction between necessary and sufficient causes.

As with a car or other mechanical device the components of the brain can be divided into those that are *necessary* for conscious experience (the frontal medial cortex, for example) and that when injured can result in disturbances in consciousness (the alien hand syndrome) but are not themselves *sufficient* to mediate consciousness. Many brain areas are necessary for consciousness, but no single one of them is sufficient in itself to mediate it. In short, no "center" for consciousness exists; rather, consciousness emerges from the activity of a presently unknown number of brain areas linked together into a network.

New technology like PET studies reveals the neurological underpinnings of attention and its more evolved sibling, consciousness. Neither results from the operation of a single brain area, nor of the brain as a whole. Rather, the brain's modules, sometimes widely separated groups of neuronal circuits, cooperatively create what none of them can do separately. The parietal and frontal areas seem particularly important, with one or the other predominating according

to the circumstances of the moment. As we will discuss at other
points throughout this book, the frontal areas are associated with the
more personal and subjective aspects of attention. But we should not
conclude that we have discovered all the relevant brain areas. Every
technology has its limitations, and PET studies are no exception. Will
further research reveal additional areas responsible for attention and
consciousness? At this point the answer to that question remains tan-
talizingly outside the limits of our knowledge.

I I

So far we have described the brain on the *macro*molecular level of how things look to the naked eye and how the whole organ can be neatly divvied up via recognizable landmarks into separate partitions. But this small organ (weighing no more than 1,500 grams, about 2 percent of total body weight) also has a microscopic structure. It is composed of two types of living cells: long, stringy *neurons* (from the Greek "to spin") and compact *glial* ("glue") cells that bind neurons together and contribute to their functioning.

In order to achieve the billions of cells comprising the mature brain, 2.5 million neurons must be generated per minute during prenatal life. All nerve cells are present at birth and, in general, a neuron that dies during a person's lifetime is not replaced. For an adult between the ages of twenty and seventy, fifty thousand neurons die or disappear each day, a rate of attrition that would seriously impair any other organized structure in the known universe. This loss over a lifetime equals less than 10 percent of the number present at birth. But such an astounding loss of neurons does not result in any noticeable loss in function since the remaining neurons can fashion new connections with other neurons to form new circuits and networks.

This capacity continues during the entire lifespan, and is the explanation for the creativity late in life of an Einstein or a Picasso.

In contrast to earlier thinking about the brain, most neuroscientists now believe the organ remains malleable throughout life. Each
thought and behavior is embedded within the circuitry of the neurons and, according to one hypothesis, neuronal activity accompanying or initiating an experience persists in the form of reverberating
neuronal circuits, which become more strongly defined with repetition. Thus habit and other forms of memory may consist of the estab-
lishment of permanent and semipermanent neuronal circuits. At least
in theory, all that we are and all that we have done could be read by
an observer capable of deciphering the connections and circuits that
have been established within our 50 billion nerve cells.

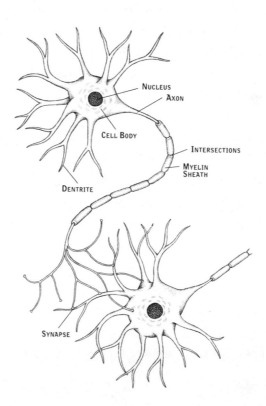

Looked at through a microscope, the neurons within the brain share a remarkably similar structure. They have been likened to a tree, with thin, sensitive-looking *dendrites* passing information *inward* toward the cell body in an arrangement like twigs or branches. Information from the cell is conveyed *outward* along a long, thin taproot-like structure that can extend several yards in length from the cortex.

The holism-localization debate about the brain function mentioned earlier is mirrored at the microscopic level by an equally intense dispute about whether the brain is best understood in terms of neurons existing as separate entities, or whether the brain consists of a dense, interweaving net of interconnected cells. This controversy has implications for the operation of the brain as a whole, for if neurons are not separate but fused together, then localization of function, which demands some degree of independence in the formation of pathways and centers, becomes impossible.

Thanks to careful observations through powerful electron microscopes we know that neurons do not actually touch but are separated by a junction, the *synapse* (a Greek term meaning "contact" or "point of juncture," chosen in 1897 by the unlikely collaboration of a brain scientist and a humanist scholar known for his expertise on Euripides). Neurons communicate with one another across synapses, establishing what Ramon y Cajal, a Spanish neuroscientist with a poetic bent, referred to as "protoplasmic kisses . . . which seem to constitute the final ecstasy of an epic love story." Well . . . not quite, unless you imagine an ethereal kiss that involves no contact.

A neuron is traditionally divided into the *cell body,* which contains the nucleus and the machinery for constructing proteins and the neuron's internal structures; an *axon,* an elongated process carrying the nerve message from the nerve cell to its neighbors; and multiple *den-*

drites, which serve as the receiving stations for nerve impulses arriving from other neurons.

Despite the obvious importance of neurons in the functioning of the brain—indeed, its activity can be described as the sum total of all neurons acting in the aggregate—they occupy only a small percentage of the number of cells in the organ. Far greater in number are the glial cells, which account for half the brain's volume and perhaps as many as nine-tenths of its cells.

Even though their numbers are large, glial cells have until recently been regarded as the orphans of neuroscience. Ignored, denigrated, or downright disowned, these ubiquitous cells have been relegated to the role of supporting structures filling in the space between neurons.

For instance, *astrocytes,* star-shaped glial cells, make intimate contact with neurons, blood vessels, and other astrocytes. It was considered that they serve as a combination food gatherer and waste recover—a kind of humble servant serving its master, the neuron.

Another class of glial cells, the *oligodendrocytes,* perform a service of a different sort. They encircle the nerve cell axon with a layer of myelin which, acting like insulation on an electric wire, increases efficiency and speeds transmission. In multiple sclerosis this insulating covering breaks down, resulting in "shorts" along the axon and a host of ensuing impairments ranging from devastating losses of sight and motion to lesser difficulties like numbness and subtle problems in muscle coordination.

Other glial cells, the *ependymal* cells, line the inner walls of the ventricles; *microglial* cells serve as scavengers that engulf intercellular debris.

While taking all of this knowledge about glia into account, some neuroscientists suggested that glial cells may also play a role in signaling and information transfer. Such speculations now seem less unorthodox in light of recent findings that the membranes of glial cells, which form such intimate connections with neurons, contain some of the same proteins found on the membrane of the nerve cells. If glial cells do turn out to play a role in transmitting information, the ante will be raised considerably on the question of the brain's complexity. To the brain's 50 billion nerve cells would be added another twenty times that number of information-transfer cells.

In any consideration of the brain at its cellular level, one thing seems certain: The brain's complexity and uniqueness has little to do with its physical composition alone. Reduced to its chemical essentials, the brain consists of the common elements carbon, hydrogen, nitrogen, and phosphorus, along with a few trace metals thrown in for good measure. Nothing in this simple blend, which can be found in all of nature, provides an explanation for the brain's power and uniqueness. For this we must look to the organization of its cells, the neurons.

Within the cerebral cortex, the thin mantle of tissue overlying the top and sides of the brain, reside an estimated 10 billion neurons linked by 1 million billion connections. Counting these connections at the rate of one connection per second would take 32 million years to complete. Even a section of the brain no bigger than a match head contains about a billion connections. Combining these into all of their various connections results in the number ten followed by millions of zeros. And to put that number into perspective, the number of positively charged particles in the whole known universe is only ten followed by eighty zeros.

Each of the brain's 50 billion nerve cells communicates by a combination of electricity and chemistry (neurotransmitters). The process depends on the actions of enzymes—proteins that regulate almost all of the chemical reactions that occur within living cells. Among other things, enzymes increase the speed of chemical reactions, sometimes by a million fold, without being permanently altered themselves.

The first of the enzymes responsible for neuron-to-neuron communication *prepares* the neuron for signaling activity. It consists of a protein that spans the width of the cell membrane so as to be in contact with both the inside of the cell, the cytoplasm, and the outside of the cell. The enzyme operates by transporting the flow of electrically charged particles known as ions—specifically, the sodium and potassium ions—across the cell membrane. This transport causes an imbalance in electrical forces, with the inside of the neuron more negatively charged than the outside. The resulting electrochemical difference is the basis for neuronal firing.

Neuroscientists usually refer to this membrane-spanning protein as the sodium-potassium pump. But this is a misleading name, since a pump is usually thought of as a stable mechanical device that remains structurally unchanged during its operation. The "enzymatic pump," in contrast, behaves more like a glob of Silly Putty, which can undergo changes in configuration.

Since the sodium-potassium pump transports three Na+ ions out of the neuron for every two K+ ions transported in, an electrical imbalance develops between the inside and the outside of the nerve cell. Since one more positively charged ion (Na+) leaves the cell than enters (K+) it, the outside becomes electrically positive while the inside becomes electrically negative. The actual electrical differential is about -0.07 volts or -70 millivolts (mV). This membrane potential, sometimes referred to as the resting potential, renders the

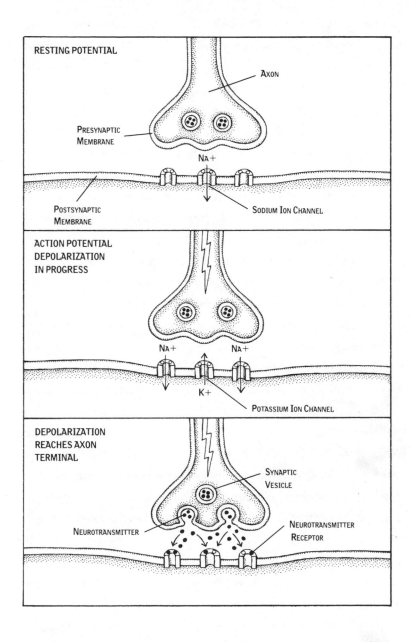

neuron ready for firing, "like a rifle that is ready and loaded," as characterized by Harvard University biologists David Dressler and Huntington Potter.

The *actual "firing"* of the neuron (the transmission of the nerve signal along the length of its axon) is produced by a tiny erosion of the -70 mV differential across the cell membrane. A local reduction in the voltage difference between inside and outside induces either an opening or a closing of special channels for sodium or potassium. Think of these *ion channels* as similar to portholes which, depending on whether they are open or closed, can admit or bar free passage of a specific ion.

The process begins with a one-thousandth-of-a-second disruption in the resting potential of the target neuron caused by the stimulatory influence of other neurons. Remember that at every microsecond of its existence, the brain is a dynamic organ in which each neuron is influencing somewhere between one thousand and ten thousand other neurons. This influence of many cells on one another creates a tiny electrical disruption on the outer surface membrane of each neuron that, if it reaches a certain threshold, suddenly alters the shape of the Na+ membrane channels. These "voltage-controlled" channels (so named since it is the change in voltage that alters their shape) open and allow Na+ ions to rush inward from the outside of the nerve cell. The massive influx of Na+ ions leads to a complete collapse of the normal -70 mV resting potential of the axon just at the point where it leads off from the cell body. This *depolarization* of the axon segment takes place in a millisecond (a thousandth of a second), at which point it rapidly reverses by means of a two-step process. The Na+ channels close while, at the same time, a second family of channels conducting potassium (K+) opens, resulting in a strong *outward* flow of K+. As the K+ ions move outward from their location of high concentration the large positive charge inside the axon begins to diminish until, a few milliseconds later, the original -70 mV resting potential across the nerve cell membrane is restored.

"Action potential" is the term neuroscientists have settled on to describe the two-step process whereby Na+ initially rushes in through its channels (depolarization) and K+ diffuses back out of the cell (repolarization).

Communication via the action potential has been compared to the chain reaction following the lighting of a fuse. The original point of excitation is propagated by means of recurring cycles of depolarization-repolarization along the length of the axon. A better analogy would be a string of dominoes connected by a thin string or wire. As one domino falls the immediately adjacent dominoes follow, and all are restored to their original order by a pull on the string.

Notable in this process is the fluidity of the ion channels. Rather than being stable structures like funnels, they are more like clouds that can swirl into different shapes and at different times permit or impede the passage of sunlight. In order to get an accurate sense of this fluidity one must think of fields of energy and force. Thus, in a way, the ancients were not completely wrong in their insistence on an evanescent influence flowing through the brain. We differ from them in our knowledge that force is material rather than ethereal.

Once an action potential has been established, the wave of depolarization travels along the length of the nerve's axon until reaching the tip, the nerve terminal. By convention two communicating neurons are referred to as the presynaptic and the postsynaptic, cells separated from each other by a tiny space, the synapse.

In order for the nerve impulse to travel across the synapse from the presynaptic to the postsynaptic cell it is transformed from an electrical signal into a chemical one.

As a first step, upon reaching the end of the presynaptic cell, the action potential loses its -70 mV charge across the membrane. This, in turn, results in the opening of channels within the membrane for calcium ions (Ca+). As calcium rushes into the interior of the axon, its higher concentration promotes a fusion along the inner wall of the presynaptic nerve cell membrane of vesicles, tiny particles containing one or more neurotransmitters, the brain's chemical messengers. Like iron filings drawn toward a magnet, the vesicles, under the influence of calcium ions, move toward the inner aspect of the membrane, fuse with it at active release zones, and eventually discharge their neurotransmitter contents into the synapse.

Once in the synapse, the neurotransmitter diffuses like a ferryboat steaming across a channel toward the "loading dock," the receptor on the membrane of the receiver cell (the postsynaptic membrane).

The receptors are the mechanisms used by neurotransmitters to permit one neuron to "talk" to another. In my book *Receptors* (1994), I made the point that the study of the receptors offers the richest, most rewarding approach to understanding how the brain works.

Briefly, receptors are large dynamic protein molecules that exist along and within the cell membrane. I describe them as "dynamic" because they can increase in number and avidity for their neurotransmitter according to circumstances. Large and prolonged intakes of certain substances, for instance, lead to an increase in the number of receptors for these substances—the basis for the withdrawal response in addiction when the receptors, deprived of their usual supply of addicting substance, "cry out" like deserted lovers for the missing chemical. Later, if the addicted person stays away from the drugs the receptors eventually die off like leaves spiraling from the branches of a tree deprived of sunlight.

Each neurotransmitter influences its own receptor independent of the action of other receptors. While some neurotransmitters decrease the voltage between the inside and the outside of the nerve cell and thus stimulate the cell into action (an excitatory neurotransmitter), others increase it and thus inhibit the cell from firing (an inhibitory neurotransmitter). At millisecond intervals the nerve cell tallies the strength of the excitatory influences, measures it against the inhibitory influences, and, based on whichever is greater, either fires off an action potential or remains quiescent. Thus a threshold on the postsynaptic cell must be reached before the nerve cell fires. This "all or nothing" response of the nerve cell resembles the on/off switch in an electrical circuit. But, in contrast to the components of an electrical circuit, each neuron is a dynamic living structure which, over its life span, measures in millisecond intervals the excitatory and inhibitory influences acting on it.

The brain as a whole can be understood as the summation of billions of interacting neurons influencing one another via the interplay of hundreds of neurotransmitters and their receptors, which in turn influence the passage of electrically charged particles across the nerve cell membrane.

Receptors fall into two categories, or what neuroscientists refer to as "superfamilies," each with its own characteristic structures and functional modes. The basis for this division is whether the receptors influence the activity of the ion channels (for sodium [Na+], potassium [K+], calcium [Ca+], and chloride [Cl-], principally) directly, or indirectly, via biochemical intermediates.

Ion channel receptors (also referred to as ligand-gated; ligand is a ten-dollar word for *chemical*) bring about changes in membrane permeability and thus govern the flow of ions through their channel. When a neurotransmitter reacts with its receptor, their interaction results in a change in the shape of the receptor so that ions can then flow across the membrane from the point of high concentration toward the point of lower concentration. It is precisely this ability that justifies the description of receptors as "dynamic" rather than conforming to the frequently proposed analogy of a "lock" that receives the neurotransmitter "key." The receptor is, in fact, more like a vibrating, exquisitely sensitive, and responsive organism that modifies its structure according to whether it's in contact with its neurotransmitter.

The second superfamily of receptors do not contain ion channels within their structures. Like plaintiffs in a lawsuit, they do not act directly but function through intermediaries, i.e., their lawyers. In this analogy lawyers correspond to special cellular proteins, the G proteins, located inside the nerve cell.

Basically, G proteins function as coupling factors that serve as links between the receptor on the outside surface of the nerve cell membrane and a vast number of interlinked cellular processes within the cell. Another analogy for the process is the spread of a rumor: one person (the neurotransmitter) starts by telling it to one person (the receptor), who later goes inside a large building and repeats it to everyone he meets. His listeners, in turn, act as "second messengers" and spread the rumor along many separate pathways.

"Cascade reactions" is the term applied to the process brought about when a ligand interacts with a second-messenger chemical, which then stimulates multiple reactions within the neuron. Some reactions are short-lived and involve such things as the synthesis of additional neurotransmitters, the number of synapses formed, or the sensitivity of receptors within the nerve cell membrane. Others are more complex and long-lasting, exerting an influence within the cell nucleus and thereby affecting the expression of genes. Thus a single event of a neurotransmitter binding to its receptor (the first-messenger level) acts within the nerve cell through second-, third-, and fourth-messenger levels to produce a dazzling cascade of independent as well as interrelated effects. As with a rumor, especially one that concerns a truth, vast and wide-ranging changes can be brought about by an amplification process: a vast explosion of interacting circuits can emanate from a single source.

In summary, neurotransmitters can act by directly altering an ion channel in the nerve cell membrane; or by G protein coupling between the receptor and the ion channel; or, finally, by G protein coupling between the receptor and a second-messenger system within the cell.

Such a tripartite system provides temporal flexibility ranging from milliseconds to decades (as in the case of memories, which can be held over a lifetime).

A neurotransmitter may also produce effects via all three mechanisms—one of the reasons for the complexity of the human brain. What's more, multiple types exist for each of the main receptors. Neuroscientists learned this by applying radioactive-labeled molecules (tags) to receptors in the membranes of nerve cells. When various drugs were then applied to the membranes some receptors of the same family took up the drug faster than others. For example, some receptors for the neurotransmitter serotonin gobbled up the drug immediately, while other serotonin receptors did so more slowly, or in some cases not at all. A classification emerged based on ranking the potency of each receptor's binding to specific drugs, and revealed that at least fourteen receptor subtypes for serotonin exist. Such research has already paid off in the development of drugs for migraine (Imitrix, which affects a specific serotonin receptor) and depression (Prozac and the family of serotonin reuptake blockers, which affect other serotonin receptors.)

The discovery of additional receptor subtypes holds promise for the development of finely "sculpted" drugs capable of acting with increasing precision in the treatment of disorders of mood, thought, and behavior. They may also prove effective in altering for the better a host of "normal" but nonetheless limiting personality characteristics like shyness, reclusiveness, and a general pessimism concerning other people and life in general.

Such variety in neurotransmitters and their receptors makes possible a marvelous variety and subtley of response in the human brain. Even within the same family of neurotransmitters different receptor subtypes make it possible for the initiation of varying cascades of chemical reactions within the interior of the neuron. This is one of the reasons why the brain can never be fully "explained." Indeed it is impossible to make either large- or small-scale predictions about exactly what will happen in the brain from one instant to another. Still more difficult is to relate it to the subjective world of our inner thoughts and emotions. But connections do exist, as we know from the effects on mental functioning brought about by drugs that influence neurotransmitters and their receptors (a subject we will have much more to say about later). The situation is similar to what confronted cartographers in Columbus's time: vast expanses were already known, others could only be guessed at, and some remained outside the limits of even the most creative imaginations.

With the action potential successfully transferred from the presynaptic to the postsynaptic cell, the stage is set for the final process in nerve cell transmission: the termination of the effect of the neurotransmitter after it has conveyed the nerve impulse across the synapse to the postsynaptic cell. This can be accomplished in either of two ways: the neurotransmitters may be recaptured by the presynaptic neuron and stored once again within the vesicle. Or, as in the case of acetylcholine, the first neurotransmitter to be discovered, the termination involves breaking down the substance into its component parts. The enzyme acetylcholinesterase cleaves acetylcholine into its original components, acetic acid and choline, in forty millionths of a second. Since the postsynaptic cell membrane recovers its resting potential within only a fraction of a second, we can infer that the synapse is capable of transmitting a thousand impulses per second. With the termination of the influence of a neurotransmitter, the pre- and postsynaptic cells return to their original state and are thus fully prepared for initiation of the next nerve impulse.

Of all the chemical substances involved in the microbiological functioning of the brain, neurotransmitters, the key elements that make rapid and long-distance communication possible throughout the brain, fall into three main categories. The simplest are comprised of single amino acids, the building blocks of protein. They are the most prevalent of the three types and may be present in upwards of 80 percent of synapses in the brain. Included here are glutamate, the most prevalent excitatory amino acid neurotransmitter in the brain, and gamma aminobutyric acid (GABA), the major inhibitory amino acid neurotransmitter.

The brain's second category of neurotransmitter also consists of amino acids, but in this case they do not act as neurotransmitters themselves but, rather, are modified within the neuron to produce the *monoamines*. This class includes the *catecholamines* (dopamine, nor-epinephrine, and epinephrine) as well as the major *indoleamine, sero-*

tonin. All of these substances are collectively referred to as biogenic amines. The *catecholamines,* despite different names and locations within the brain, resemble one another so closely that one has to have some training in chemistry or stare long and hard at their chemical formulas in order to distinguish them.

As another distinguishing feature they are organized into discrete nuclei located in the brain stem that project upward toward cortical and subcortical targets.

Rounding out the biogenic class is *acetylcholine.* Its discoverer, Otto Loewi, came upon a fundamental insight about its existence in a dream which he related in a delightful sketch that is worthy of this brief digression:

The night before Easter Sunday of that year [1920] I awoke, turned on the light, and jotted down a few notes on a tiny slip of thin paper. Then I fell asleep again. It occurred to me at six o'clock in the morning that during the night I had written down something most important, but I was unable to decipher the scrawl. The next night at three o'clock the idea returned. It was the design of an experiment to determine whether or not the hypotheses of chemical transmission that I had uttered seventeen years ago was correct. I got up immediately, went to the laboratory, and performed a simple experiment on a frog heart according to the nocturnal design. . . . These results unequivocally proved that the nerves do not influence the heart directly but liberate from their terminals specific chemical substances which, in their turn, cause the well known modifications of the function of the heart characteristic of the stimulation of its nerves.

Despite the fact that only a small percentage of neurons employ monoamines as neurotransmitters, most of the efforts up till now to understand the chemical nature of the brain in health and disease have concentrated on these chemicals. Indeed, the first theory about the chemical basis of depression postulated that the illness resulted from a deficiency of monoamines at key synapses; the treatment proposed involved the administration of drugs that increased the synaptic availability of monoamines. This explanation, while initially promising, has turned out to be overly simplistic.

The monoamine dopamine has been the focus of research aimed at curing schizophrenia, and at the moment different subtypes of the dopamine receptor are the targets of the most effective drugs against the disease. While their success suggests that dopaminergic pathways regulate in some way the neuronal circuits that cause the illness, this isn't the same thing as saying that schizophrenia is *caused* by a primary dysfunction in dopamine neurons or dopamine receptors. Such complex conditions are unlikely to result from a disturbance in a single neurotransmitter or its receptor.

Only one illness has so far been definitely linked with a deficiency of a specific neurotransmitter. Parkinson's disease, marked by a tremor and slowed voluntary movement, results from a selective loss of dopamine-containing neurons in a nucleus in the midbrain. Since this correlation is one of the most famous discoveries in the history of neuroscience, it's worth taking a moment to develop it in more detail.

Three nuclei contain cell bodies of dopamine-producing neurons. Two of these are in the brain stem, and the third is located farther up in the hypothalamus. Located in the brain stem, the *substantia nigra*—affected in Parkinson's—projects primarily to the corpus striatum, composed of the basal ganglia nuclei, the caudate, and the putamen.

As we discussed earlier, the basal ganglia mediate automatic and accessory movements. Thus, the loss of dopamine to this area and the resulting degeneration of the dopamine pathways from substantia nigra to corpus striatum induces in the afflicted person a slow, labored gait, loss of the natural swing of the arms while walking, and other motor disturbances. A similar picture results from the use of antipsychotic drugs, which are given to block the action of dopamine at its receptor. (Such drugs are called "antagonists.") Indeed, even a skilled neurologist cannot always distinguish a patient suffering from Parkinson's Disease from one showing the side effects induced by an antipsychotic drug.

The *ventral tegmental* dopamine-producing neurons project to the limbic system and parts of the cerebral cortical structures that are important in the experience and expression of emotion. Antipsychotic drugs are believed to work by antagonizing the actions of dopamine in this system; the Parkinson-like effects mentioned above are undesirable side effects caused by blocking the pathway leading from the substantia nigra to the corpus striatum.

The newest antipsychotic drugs specifically target the dopamine pathways leading to the limbic and cortical regions while having no effect on the pathways from substantia nigra to corpus striatum. Such drugs make possible fine, almost microprecise distinctions in treatment. For instance, a patient of mine with Parkinson's disease improved dramatically on a drug that supplied the missing dopamine in the pathway from the substantia nigra. Although his movements loosened up, and his tremor stopped, he also experienced visual hallucinations and paranoid fears that mysterious "others" were talking about him. These symptoms of psychosis resulted from the undesirable effect of the administered dopa (which is transformed in the brain to the neurotransmitter dopamine) on the circuit going from ventral tegmental neurons up to the limbic system. The psychosis abated when I gave him the antipsychotic drug Clozapine, which selectively blocks dopamine's actions in the limbic areas while leaving it free to act in the corpus striatum.

Other monoamine pathways involve projection systems from the brain stem upward toward different parts of the forebrain. *Noradrenaline* (also called norepinephrine) projects from a small nucleus called the *locus coeruleus,* which is composed of about twelve thousand large neurons on each side of the brain. It projects upward to more brain areas than any of the other nuclei. Its neurons are activated in states of heightened vigilance, hence its probable role in anxiety states, sleep disorders, and some aspects of mental disorders, such as schizophrenia and manic depression. Many of the drugs for these disorders appear to work by influencing norepinephrine availability or utilization.

Serotonin projects from the dorsal and ventral raphe. Our knowledge of this neurotransmitter and its receptors has grown significantly during the past decade. Its major receptor subtypes govern matters as diverse as migraine headache and depression. Drugs that affect the 5-HT1A serotonin receptor lessen anxiety without, as usually happens, inducing drowsiness. Interestingly, the antianxiety effect takes weeks to occur—an indication that sometimes anxiety relief may require prolonged receptor modification. Another serotonin receptor, the 5-HT1D receptor, is widely distributed in the brain, and its blockage by the drug sumatriptan leads to the prompt relief of migraine. The drug has no effect at other serotonin receptors, an example of how different each of the serotonin receptors is from all others. Blockage of a third type of receptor, the 5-HT2, also relieves migraine, but by a completely different mechanism.

Special drugs that prevent the reuptake of serotonin from the synapse produce the most efficient and successful antidepressant effect of any pharmaceutical treatment in history. (Side effects are mild in comparison with earlier antidepressants aimed at affecting the dopamine or norepinephrine pathways). Included in this category is Prozac, a psychiatric drug that has exerted a powerful social and cultural impact on American society. Its truly astonishing effects on deep-seated and prolonged depressions have revolutionized our ideas about emotions and thought. If a person can begin to feel better about himself or herself as a result of a chemical that modifies the action of a brain neurotransmitter, even in situations when no outward change has taken place in that person's day-to-day existence, what does that imply about the biological foundation for our inner life? At the very least it supports what neuroscientists have been suggesting over the past three decades: All things mental are embedded within the chemistry and neuronal circuitry of the brain. We will say more about this later but for now it's sufficient to point out that panic disorders, anxiety, depression, and obsessive-compulsive disorder are no longer looked upon as the result of mysterious and controversial psychological dysfunctions, but the outer manifestations of intrinsic brain malfunctions.

Acetylcholine, whose function was discovered by Loewi after his prophetic dream, interacts with multiple receptors. One of these, the nicotinic receptor, binds the nicotine in tobacco. When inhaled, tobacco smoke delivers the nicotine to the lungs and then on via the blood stream to the brain, where it binds to its own receptor. This linkage of acetylcholine to its receptor is especially strong within areas of the limbic system involved in the pleasure response—the reason smokers have such difficulties breaking their habit. Acetylcholine also works at the junction between nerves and muscles.

When the chemical is released from a nerve ending it diffuses across the synaptic junction and is taken up by acetylcholine receptors on the muscle fibers. The resulting bond between neurotransmitter and receptor results in muscle movement. This process can be interfered with by compounds such as curare, a herbal poison employed for centuries by South American Indians. Curare works by competing with acetylcholine for its receptor and thereby inhibiting the normal depolarization that produces muscle movement. Thus, the victim is not only paralyzed but asphyxiated thanks to blockage of the muscles responsible for breathing.

As we have discussed earlier, after a neurotransmitter and its receptor have reacted, the process must be brought to a halt, which is accomplished either by destruction of the neurotransmitter and recycling of its chemical constituents, or by a so-called reuptake system, whereby the neurotransmitter is recaptured and stored once again within the vesicle. In the case of acetylcholine, the process involves a breakdown brought about by the enzyme acetylcholinesterase, which cleaves the neurotransmitter back to its original chemical building blocks. This process can be interfered with by compounds responsible for some of the worst horrors of twentieth-century warfare. Nerve gases, such as the deadly Sarin released into the subway system in Tokyo in March 1995, form irreversible bonds with anticholinesterase, thus inhibiting the enzymes' ability to break down acetylcholine in the synapse. The resulting buildup of acetylcholine brings on symptoms experienced by many of the subway victims: dimming of vision, intense sweating, vomiting, convulsions and, if treatment isn't available, death from paralysis of respiratory muscles overstimulated by excess acetylcholine.

Other interferences with the acetylcholine receptor can produce a range of effects from the horrifying to the merly inconvenient. Botulinum toxin, produced by a spore-forming bacteria contaminating home-canned foods, results in the nearly always fatal botulism marked by symptoms produced by blocking the delivery of acetylcholine to receptors *outside* the brain at the junction of nerves and muscles and in the autonomic nervous system. Difficulty chewing, swallowing, and breathing lead inexorably to paralysis and death. *Within* the brain, the most common problem comes from drugs that occupy the acetylcholine receptor site but do not activate it (anticholinergic). In some instances this can lead to delirium, confusion, memory loss, and symptoms of a toxic psychosis. More often, the anticholinergic effect is less serious and expressed solely by acetylcholine receptors outside the brain in the peripheral nervous system. This includes dryness in the mouth and throat secondary to the drug's inhibiting effect on salivation and mucus production. (These effects are deliberately taken advantage of in "cold" remedies, which by design include anticholinergic drugs.) Within the brain, the anticholinergic effects of memory loss and incipient delirium can be reversed by drugs that interfere with the (acetylcholinesterase) breakdown of acetylcholine. These chemicals have been tried, but with little success, as a means to reverse the memory loss in some cases of early Alzheimer's disease, thought to be at least partly caused by low levels of functioning acetylcholine in key brain areas.

The final class of neurotransmitters are the *neuropeptides*. These are small molecules, sometimes comprising just a few amino acids, with an irregular distribution in the brain: Some are found in very restricted brain areas, while others can be found throughout the brain. They may also diffuse freely and affect receptors at some distance from the neuron that releases them. (They share this property with hormones that diffuse freely and exert an influence at great distances.) Neuropeptides exist not only in the brain but in organs like the lung, the stomach, and the sex organs—a hint that overly rigid distinctions should not be made between the brain and the rest of the body. As noted, anticholinergic drugs acting at various places in the body can produce unpleasant and disturbing side effects that make normal perception, thinking, and feeling almost impossible. Think back to the last time you had a really bad case of the flu—particularly one with a lot of headache, fever, and malaise. You recognized, along with everyone acquainted with you, that you were not "yourself." And yet the majority of your symptoms resulted from the illness's effects elsewhere in your body than in your brain. Many of these effects were triggered by neuropeptides. Disturbances in neuropeptides, along with other neurotransmitters, underlie many of the symptoms of psychiatric illness. It is likely that over the next decade or so mental illnesses will be defined in terms of neurotransmitter imbalances within areas of the brain involved in emotional processing, with medications designed to target the specific receptors affected. Although much of the emphasis in past research has been on dopamine, the neurotransmitters glutamate and gamma aminobutyric acid (GABA) are present within the brain in much larger amounts. We will say more later about the chemical modification of personality, behavior, and feelings.

III

So far we have explored the brain at two levels: its major demarcations and centers, and its 50 billion neurons which communicate by means of neurotransmitters acting across synapses. It is time to drop down one additional level:

Brain cells, like every other cell in the human body, contain a genetic code written out in the form of extended molecules, the chromosomes. But only a fraction of all the genes on the chromosomes are expressed within any cell. This selective expression of genes and the proteins they code for determines how that cell will function. The brain is no exception to this rule: it is specialized for information transfer.

DNA, the physical structure of heredity, differs not at all from one species to another. Chemically it's impossible to distinguish between cat DNA, horse DNA, and human DNA. The difference between a frog and a prince lies in the way the four chemical components in DNA are arranged. This quartet of chemicals, or nucleotide bases, to employ the technical term for them, have scientific names—guanine, cytosine, thymine, and adenine—but they are usually identified as G, C, T, and A. Every life structure and process can be expressed in some sequence of these four letters. And tiny variations can account for enormous differences. For instance, humans differ from chimpanzees by about one percent of the three billion or so DNA bases in their genes. While this may seem like a small amount, one percent of three billion comes to thirty million differences between ourselves and our closest relatives. How many of these differences are meaningful? Probably no more than 1 percent are of any consequence in explaining human-chimp differences. And so far scientists haven't the slightest idea about the number and location of the genes responsible for brain size, intelligence, or other aspects of brain function.

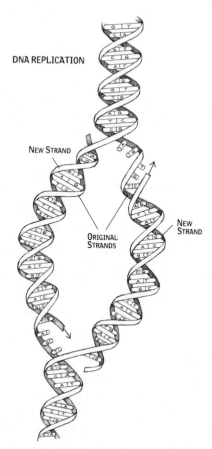

DNA is often compared to a twisted rope ladder with the As, Gs, Ts, and Cs arranged as the rungs of the ladder. Each nucleotide is joined end to end with its complement (A joins only with T and G only with C). The two strands of the rope ladder wind around and around each other like an endless circular stairway. Millions of As, Ts, Gs, and Cs occur along each of the two strands. This two-stranded coil of DNA is known as a chromosome. Each cell in the body contains forty-six or twenty-three pairs of these chromosomal rope ladders with each chromosome containing several thousand genes located at corresponding points along their length. The order of the nucleotides in a given gene specifies the formula for one of the 100,000 proteins found in the human body. The possible permutations are so large that it's estimated that the entire human race born so far represents less than 1 percent of the potential nucleotide arrangements.

At first scientists doubted that DNA alone could provide the basis for heredity because of the apparent simplicity of its chemical composition (consisting of only four subunits). But that attitude failed to take into account two key features of DNA: its helical structure and the strong attraction of As, Ts, Gs, and Cs. The helical shape facilitates self-copying. During cell division the helices unzip, separating each chromosome into separate strands. This leaves the nucleotide bases along each strand shorn of their complement. But within a thousandth of a second the single strand once again becomes two thanks to the complementary binding of unattached nucleotides. Each linear sequence of three nucleotides specifies a single amino acid, the small molecules that join together to form proteins.

If the process stopped here, DNA would be caught up in a endless round of self-replication but deprived of any means of influencing events outside the nucleus of the cell. To accomplish this, the information in DNA, coded by means of the linear sequence of its nucleotides, is transcribed to an RNA strand that breaks free and exits the nucleus. Since RNA contains a complementary base pairing to the DNA from which it originated—its sequence provides exact information about the sequence in the DNA template—all of the genetic information in the DNA can be deciphered via the message coded in the nucleotide sequence of RNA.

The messenger RNA (mRNA) differs from DNA in one important way: it is more telegraphic. Just as a telegram omits words unnecessary to the basic message, mRNA eliminates nucleotide sequences that do not seem to encode any information. For reasons no one understands, less than 1 percent of human DNA carries information that is actually used for the construction of proteins; the rest exists in the form of short repetitive sequences that do not code for anything. (Of 3 billion base pairs of DNA there are about 100,000 genes; 30,000 of these are expressed in the brain.) The information-conveying units—called *exons*, since this information is *exported* from the cell nucleus—are interrupted by introns, the noncoding sequences. The inclusion of tandem repeats of random DNA on the chromosome may serve some presently unknown function such as stabilizing DNA's structure. In any case, during a messenger RNA replication this seemingly useless *non*information is removed by enzymes within the nucleus and the exons are spliced together and exported from the nucleus in the form of mRNA.

Once it reaches the cytoplasm outside the nucleus, the mRNA binds to ribosomes, particles that translate the message from mRNA into amino acids that, in combination, make up proteins. Once released from the ribosomes, the amino acids bind to various chemical groups (sugar, phosphate, etc.) to form bonds that bestow such identifying characteristics as three-dimensional structure, chemical

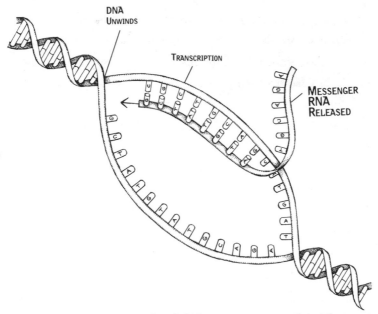

reaction patterns, and solubility in water or fat. The variety of functions performed by different cells in the body results from the number and type of proteins formed. Although each cell in the body contains the same chromosome pattern, the same DNA sequences, and thus the same genes, only a tiny fraction of all genes are expressed in any given cell type. (This fact is the basis for the frequent science-fiction scenario whereby an entire human being is built up from only one cell by stimulating that cell to multiply a few times and then turning on genes in different cells so as to produce all of the body's cells and organs.) Thus, although a skin cell and a neuron contain the same DNA, many of the genes that are actively transcribed and transferred from the nucleus in the neuron are not expressed in the skin cell. Each body cell represents some aspect of information transfer from the genome (the whole complement of genes contained in the DNA) to the cytoplasm, where each cell's identifying and unique protein structure is encoded.

With brain cells the process of information transfer takes on a self-reflective aspect: the brain cell represents the essence of information transfer, and indeed exists for no other purpose at every level of its functioning, from actions and feelings at the macroscopic level to the swirl of neurotransmitters at the molecular level. From this perspective, inherited forms of normal and abnormal brain functioning are a reflection of either "correct" or "incorrect" transfers of information somewhere in the path from DNA to protein.

For instance, Huntington's disease, which killed folksinger Woody Guthrie, is caused by means of a mutation in one gene on the fourth of the forty-six human chromosomes. Although its exact effect is unknown, it's likely that the altered gene produces a chemical toxic to the specific cells destroyed in Huntington's. Treatment in the future could involve identifying and neutralizing that toxin or reversing the process and using the toxin as a clue to work backward to discover the mutation of DNA that produced it.

On the horizon are discoveries of genes that render a person more or less likely to develop a neuropsychiatric illness. Except in rare instances, genetic "loading" for a particular illness won't always guarantee its development, and greater or lesser degrees of vulnerability will exist in different individuals. Following the identification of the gene responsible for a given illness, neuroscientists will turn their attention to the resultant structural and functional properties conferred on the brains of affected individuals. In some instances this will involve disturbances in specific neurotransmitters or their interactions with one another. Neurochemistry and genetics are turning out to be more important than anatomy.

However rewarding such research promises to be, the strict

assignments of neuropsychiatric illnesses to specific genes is likely to be more the exception than the rule. For one thing, the unfolding of human personality, normal or otherwise, involves more than a simple expression of information from a genetic blueprint. In addition defining many disorders of behavior involves subjective judgments of the sort that aren't required for diagnosing standard medical illnesses. Just as one person's terrorist is another person's patriot, some would consider a depressive personality as nothing more serious than an instance of somber reflectiveness. Genetic studies have been of limited help where such distinctions are concerned.

For instance, genetic predisposition among the Amish for bipolar disorder (manic depression) frequently involves a single genetic locus on chromosome 11. But not all the Amish with the disease have this marker, suggesting that either different forms of the illness exist, or that different genetic markers can code for the same illness. What will be required to be able to make any correlation between genetics and neuropsychiatric conditions will be not only the identification of the genetic abnormalities predisposing to those illnesses but also the investigation of how different environments influence the genes. From this research will come new treatments aimed at altering the genes or, more likely, neutralizing through drugs the gene products responsible for the illness. The details of how this will be done involve a lot more neurobiology than we need go into and, in any case, are secondary to my main point: brain function and dysfunction can be understood in terms of information transfer.

To understand fully this brain-information transfer link will require additional discoveries and refinements in our knowledge of the brain's basic molecular biology. By the year 2005, and at an estimated cost of $3 billion, scientists hope to have localized on the human chromosome all of the estimated 100,000 human genes. Their final goal? To spell out the entire message conveyed by 3 billion chemical code letters in the human genome. If they are successful, their results will be of particular significance to brain research, since many brain diseases are now known to be inherited. But knowing the genetic basis for a brain disorder may still leave us without a means of curing or even significantly influencing the disease.

While a neurology resident several years ago I encountered Randy, a ten-year-old mentally retarded boy who had to be restrained in order to prevent him from committing acts of self-mutilation. At this young age he had already bitten off the ends of his fingers and inflicted such damage to his lips that his doctors considered removing his teeth in order to prevent additional harm. Randy suffered from Lesch-Nyhan syndrome. At the time nobody knew the cause of this bizarre condition, but in the intervening years scientists have identified the defective gene along with its specific DNA sequence abnormalities, and even the defective gene product. Yet even armed with this detailed genetic and molecular information, doctors have no idea why, precisely, patients like Randy mutilate themselves. Genes cannot be understood in isolation but only in the context of brain structure and function.

Whatever the limitations of current research, neuroscientists *are* making good progress in unraveling the interrelationships of genes to neuropsychiatric disorders. Genetic discoveries over the next decade will change our ideas about disorders of mood (depression and mania), anxiety (panic, phobia, obsession-compulsion), and thought (schizophrenia)—the three major classes of inherited mental illness. Rather than defining single diseases, each of these descriptive categories will likely be found to consist of genetically distinct but overlapping disorders. Moreover, specific genetic mechanisms will probably be discovered to underlie the distinguishing features of each of the variations of these illnesses.

Genetic research on neuropsychiatric illnesses like Alzheimer's disease point to what can be expected in the future. A mutation in gene coding on chromosome 14 is presently associated with up to 90 percent of cases of Alzheimer's disease beginning at or before sixty years of age, and conforms to inherited patterns. But in instances where the Alzheimer's starts later, the cause is thought to be an environmental trigger. Thus, Alzheimer's is not a distinct illness, as previously believed, but comprises a spectrum of disorders of varying severity occurring at different times and under differing conditions.

Currently more than forty disorders of the brain, spinal cord, and peripheral nervous system are associated with gene mutations. Recent research has laid bare the molecular nature of some of these genetic mutations:

A defective gene on chromosome 5 produces an alteration in the encoding of one subunit of the receptor for the inhibitory neurotransmitter glycine. Individuals with this defective gene respond to loud noises or someone's touching them with severe spasms and muscle rigidity. In infants this tendency, called hyperekplexia, can lead to death from apnea (a stoppage in breathing). Adults afflicted with the disorder are susceptible to serious falls. While hyperekplexia can be successfully treated with a benzodiazepine drug, the nature of the disorder remained mysterious until the discovery of the encoding problem on chromosome 5. "It is like finding a needle in a haystack—one base pair of change in three billion," according to John Wasmuth, director of the research team at the University of California in Irvine, a member of the international team that uncovered the world's first instance of a disease linked to a defect in a *single* neurotransmitter receptor.

The "fragile X" syndrome, the most common inherited form of mental retardation, derives its name from the appearance within cell culture of a break or gap near the end of the X chromosome of an affected individual. The site of the mutation responsible for this disorder is a small region of the X chromosome containing a gene identified as FMR1. This gene is variable in length and contains a repeat sequence of the nucleotides cytosine-guanine-guanine (CGG). In normal cases, the gene contains about thirty CGG repeats (known as amplifications), with a range of between five and fifty. "Fragile X" syndrome corresponds to a photocopy machine that just won't shut off and produces extra copies of CGG, ranging from two hundred to two thousand.

To date Huntington's disease is the best characterized and most disabling brain disease resulting from nucleotide amplifications. On chromosome 4 the normal cytosine-adenine-guanine repetition varies from 9 to 37 copies. In those afflicted with Huntington's the length ranges from 37 to 121, copies with the larger number associated with an earlier onset and greater severity of the illness. Dissimilar brain diseases apparently share similar mechanisms of expression. Although Huntington's and "fragile X" syndrome, for instance, are marked by different unstable repeat sequences in DNA, in both diseases the more severe the illness, the more unstable the sequence.

Huntington's disease is a model for how our understanding of other disease will enfold when the Human Genome Project has completed its work. At the moment Huntington's can now be diagnosed before birth by genetic testing of fetal cells obtained at amniocente-

sis. PET scans of the unaffected children of Huntington's disease sufferers can also be employed to identify which ones are likely to come
down with the illness. But since Huntington's is presently untreatable
and invariably fatal, the employment of tests for anything other than
prenatal screening raises delicate ethical questions. Who has a right to
know whether a person carries the gene for Huntington's? Suppose
one member of a twin pair wants to be tested but the other does not?
(Since twins share identical chromosomes, a positive test for one
member virtually assures that the other is similarly affected.)

Such determinations are complicated by the fact that genetically
based brain diseases differ markedly in their expression. In instances
of complete *penetrance* of the disorder, "Everybody who's got the
gene is going to have the disease. And they're going to have it in a
devastating fashion," said Albert R. Jonsen, chairman of the Department of Medical History and Genetics at the University of Washington. But such situations are relatively rare when it comes to genetic
diseases.

More usual are diseases like "fragile X" that vary in their expression. One person may inherit the most serious form of the illness
while another may inherit so mild a form that he or she has no inkling
of its presence. Thus the genetic diagnosis of brain disease is likely to
remain of only limited value, since tests available in the foreseeable
future will measure only a person's *susceptibility* to a disease rather
than determining with precision who will get the disease and indi-
cating the seriousness of the disorder.

Other genetic tests may influence our attitudes toward social and
legal issues involving certain forms of violent and criminal behavior.
In October 1993, scientists in the Netherlands reported their
research on several mentally retarded males given to sudden impul-

sive aggressive outbursts. They discovered a genetic defect on a region of the X chromosome near genes known to encode for monoamine oxidases A and B (MAOA, MAOB), two enzymes involved in the breakdown of the neurotransmitters serotonin, dopamine, and noradrenaline. Their subjects had below-normal levels of MAOA, which leads to an alteration in the processing and breakdown of these three neurotransmitters. Their findings are in line with previous studies showing reduced central serotonin function in certain people in the general population given to sudden impulsive aggression. So far no one knows whether impulsive aggression in these men is a reflection of a complete or only partial deficiency of MAOA. And the distinction is an important one, since a complete loss of MAOA would be consistent with a fully developed gene *disease* while a partial deficiency would imply only a *susceptibility*. In either case, treatments for this disorder, termed "abnormal behavior associated with a point mutation in the structural gene for monoamine oxidase A," will await neuroscientists' determination of the frequency of MAOA deficiency in the general population as well as the various neurochemical alterations brought on by the selective MAOA deficiency.

In this instance, the hope is that a serious brain disease, whose sufferers may potentially affect many people, will yield to a chemical approach, effectively eliminating the genetic predisposition toward a specific form of impulsive violence. Similar genetic discoveries and subsequent ethical quandaries are likely for other neuropsychiatric disorders since, at least in the near term, scientists' capacities to diagnose these ravaging diseases will exceed their capacities to treat or cure them.

Gene therapy might provide one future approach toward the cure of inherited brain diseases. A model for how this treatment might work comes from recent research on lupus (systemic lupus erythematosus). In mice the illness, an inflammatory disorder affecting many parts of the body including joints, skin, blood vessels, and the brain, results from a defect in a gene called Fas. If embryos from mice that have inherited two copies of the flawed gene are removed during pregnancy and a normal Fas gene is inserted into the embryos, the pups don't develop lupus. Moreover, the normal Fas gene proceeds to produce normal rather than lupus-related protein products. The end result is a healthy mouse.

Genetic disease affecting the human brain are, of course, more complicated than a generalized inflammatory disease in a mouse. With the exception of illnesses like hyperekplexia, other brain diseases almost certainly affect many neurotransmitters and are thus unlikely to result from a single gene locus. But with additional knowledge may come an increasingly targeted approach in which normal genes are inserted to correct for the effects of defective ones. Important questions must be answered in the meantime, however. Which is the best method to deliver the gene? Should genetically modified cells be implanted, or should the neurons be infected directly? How long can an inserted gene continue to express itself via the protein that it codes for? Another method for expressing desired genetic effects in the brain might involve modifying a cell elsewhere in the body by placing it in a culture medium and then transplanting it into the brain where it could function as a living "mini pump." In this way genetic modifications could be brought about without the need for establishing or altering synapses.

Whatever the methods employed, the brain will be using the corrected genes to reverse or overcome the effects of the inherited defective ones. But at this point no one can be certain gene therapy aimed at correcting inherited brain disease will represent a major breakthrough or a costly and ultimately time-consuming distraction.

IV

Most of what we know about the brain has come from the meticulous examination of the effects of injuries or illnesses. Typically, a neurologist correlates what is observed about the affected patient during his illness with changes in the brain discovered during an autopsy examination. The process is very much like the art of the detective, a comparison not lost on Sir Arthur Conan Doyle, who based Sherlock Holmes on one of the most acute neurologic diagnosticians Doyle encountered during his medical training years at Edinburgh.

As an example of the neuroscientist as sleuth consider one Hugh Cairns, an English neurosurgeon who, in 1940, encountered a patient who never spoke unless spoken to, and then only occasionally to answer questions in whispered monosyllables. He would follow Cairns as he walked about the hospital room and look steadily at him if he sat down by the bedside. Tests carried out by Cairns revealed a cyst pressing on the walls of the third ventricle located deep within and toward the midline of the brain. During surgery the cyst was aspirated, resulting in the disappearance of the patient's strange demeanor and behavior. After his recovery the patient could not recall anything that had happened during his illness.

Cairns's patient had akinetic mutism, a condition defined as "a state of unresponsiveness to the environment with extreme reluctance to perform even elementary motor activities despite the absence of paralysis." When first encountered, an individual suffering from this bizarre disorder is often suspected of feigning the illness, and in fact many of its victims are mistakenly diagnosed as suffering from a psychiatric disturbance such as catatonia. But the problem is, in fact, caused by damage to the cingulate area, located just below the motor cortex and hidden within the commissure dividing the left and right hemispheres. A PET scan of a patient with akinetic mutism will reveal damage in that area, and usually on both sides of the brain. Based on studies of patients with akinetic mutism and normal individuals while measuring effortful mental concentration, neuroscientists now believe the anterior cingulate is important in forming and maintaining information about things in their absence.

Let me provide another example of neurological sleuthing taken from a real patient encountered at the UCLA School of Medicine.

At age fifty-six Jonathan Plume began experiencing difficulties finding his way about in familiar places and in understanding what he was reading. A year or so later he developed additional difficulties with writing and in performing simple calculations like setting forth correct amounts of money in payment in restaurants and stores. Finally, eight years after the start of his difficulties, Jonathan could no longer trust himself to come up with the correct words to make his meaning plain. At this point he sought the help of a neurologist.

To the untrained observer Jonathan seemed not that much different from any other man of sixty-four with the same education and life experiences. But careful listening to his speech patterns revealed short pauses marking his attempts to come up with appropriate words. Frequently his final choice of word contained a slight but important alteration such as *tea* when he meant *see, vest* when he meant *west*. He could repeat back simple sentences spoken to him and comprehend a series of instructions. He failed utterly when asked to identify simple objects (a comb, a pen) but improved dramatically when offered the opportunity of touching the objects. Reading and writing were severely impaired. Most dramatic and distinguishing was a constellation of difficulties, named after Josef Gerstmann, the neurologist who discovered it in 1924, that Jonathan suffered.

Sufferers from Gerstmann's syndrome are unable to name their own fingers or to indicate the identity of a particular digit when asked. They have equal difficulty identifying the fingers of other people. Rarely do those with Gerstmann's syndrome complain about their impairment, since the need for such identifications occurs rarely except during wedding ceremonies or ring fittings. In addition the affected person confuses right from left, loses the ability to calculate, and cannot write. Examination of the brains of persons with Gerstmann's syndrome reveal in most instances some disease process (marked by a lesion) in a specific portion of the parietal lobe of the left hemisphere.

During Jonathan's neurological examination he also had difficulty moving his gaze from one target to another, and when shown an array of objects he always missed one or more of them. When asked to reach out and touch an object, he missed it by as much as several inches. This combination of behaviors is also familiar to clinical neurologists. Known as Balint's syndrome, it occurs secondary to brain damage in *both* hemispheres at the junction between the parietal lobe and the visual center in the occipital lobe directly to the rear.

A magnetic resonance imaging (MRI) exam of Jonathan revealed atrophy most prominent in the parietal-occipital areas on both sides of the brain. Another test showed a decrease in blood flow in these areas.

Over the next two years Jonathan's condition worsened. He depended exclusively on touch in order to identify common objects around him. Visual hallucinations and agitation finally led to his placement in a nursing home, where he died. Autopsy confirmed the loss of tissue in the posterior parts of the brain.

Jonathan's sad illness illustrates the correspondence that exists between brain disease and behavioral abnormalities. The investigation starts after either the patient or the patient's relatives or friends observe something out of the ordinary about what the patient says or does. The neurologist then combines this historical information with a specialized examination aimed at uncovering signs of brain disease. These preliminary investigations are then correlated with findings from special tests like MRI and PET scans. In most instances the dysfunction is a limited one. As with Jonathan, the brain does not suffer a total breakdown, at least initially, but specialized operations are affected. As I described in considerable detail in my book *The Modular Brain (1994)*, the brain is best thought of as composed of many interacting though separate and distinctive modules. While integrated experience depends on the integration of these modules, any of them can malfunction yet leave other equally complex operations intact.

Basic mental control mechanisms such as awareness, willed movement, and consciousness require the normal functioning of certain areas such as the brain stem (wakefulness) and cerebral cortex (language, the expression of will via movement, etc.) but no one of them is sufficient in itself to govern such functions independently. In short, there is no Papal module that oversees and controls all the others. Yet we experience ourselves as unified and not modular; we feel essentially, though not entirely, integrated. So far even our most insightful thinkers have failed to provide an explanation of how our sense of ourselves as a unity can evolve out of the operation of many separate components, each of which depends on and influences the operation of the others. (Multiple personalities and certain mental illnesses marked by a splitting off of conscious awareness, which are classified as *dissociative* disorders, illustrate the high price that is exacted when the unity of the personality is splintered.)

As a final example of neurological sleuthing let me introduce you to a patient of my own. When I first saw Gail in a hospital emergency room she was frightened and puzzled. This thirty-three-year-old mother of two and housewife complained of a severe headache, but something else was bothering her even more. She told me that an hour earlier she had been in a store and was about to write a check to cover her purchases. As she began to prepare the check she couldn't write the name of the store or the amount she owed. She "knew what [she] wanted to write but just couldn't get [her] brain to write it." Embarrassed and alarmed she signed the check, asked the clerk to fill in all of the other information, went to her car, and began the short drive home. Within a few minutes Gail was hit with a tremendous headache severe enough to force her to pull to the side of the road. Sunlight increased her headache; she closed her eyes in order to gain some relief from the escalating intensity of the pain. She stretched across the front seat, overcome with dizziness and nausea. A policeman who pulled over to check on the problem summoned an ambulance to take her to the nearest hospital. When I was called in for consultation the headache had started to remit. Most puzzling to her, and to me as well, was what she had experienced in the store. But that problem, too, had remitted since Gail no longer exhibited any abnormalities during informal testing of her reading and writing abilities.

The sudden onset of a severe headache along with accompanying nausea and vomiting are hallmarks of both the most serious and most trivial of illnesses. In the former case they may announce ruptures of aneurysms—bulges in the weakened walls of blood vessels. The blood pours out of the vessel and irritates pain-sensitive coverings of the brain. If the bleeding doesn't stop, the patient dies. If it does stop (the vessel goes into spasm), the patient may still die, since the slightest disturbance, such as a rise in blood pressure brought on by excitement, may overcome the spasm and restart the bleeding.

Obviously a subarachnoid hemorrhage is not a diagnosis that either the patient or the doctor can afford to miss. A CAT scan and spinal tap (both methods of detecting bleeding) of Gail turned out negative. Armed with this information I felt confident in telling her she had nothing to worry about and that she had experienced a particularly severe and unusual variation of an illness that had plagued her since childhood: migraine headache.

Although migraine usually involves a headache accompanied by some visual disturbances, it can take more complicated and worrisome forms. With Gail the headache was preceded by a compromise of the blood supply to one or more areas involved in the formulation of written words. As this narrowing of the blood vessels started to diminish, the pounding headache came on, the effect of an overly compensatory blood vessel enlargement. In time that, too, remitted, and the headache ceased, leaving Gail feeling "washed out but happy to hear that it was only [her] migraine."

Notice that each of these patients initially represented a point along a continuum, with a severe brain disorder at one end (akinetic mutism), extending to a more subtle, less serious disorder (Jonathan Plume) in the middle and, finally, to Gail, afflicted with the common and relatively harmless condition of migraine at the other end. In each instance some disorder of thought, emotion, or behavior resulted from damage to a particular part of the brain. Neither the problems experienced by the patients nor the speed of their progression necessarily distinguished the malignant from the relatively benign. (Gail lost her ability to speak and write almost instantaneously, whereas in the other two instances the effects were more gradual.) Rather, the seriousness of the conditions depended principally on whether the damage was permanent, as with Jonathan Plume, or whether the relevant brain areas were only momentarily affected, as with Cairns's patient and Gail.

Until recently new knowledge about the brain depended on the ability of neurologists to correlate symptoms and mental changes in patients like Cairns's and Jonathan, who had specific damage to various parts of their brains. While there is no denying the helpfulness of assigning behavioral impairments to brain lesions in order to learn more about the brain's organization and functioning, this grim approach has its limits. Brain damage doesn't respect neat anatomical landmarks but typically also involves nearby areas. Only so much can be concluded about the normal brain on the basis of studying a diseased one.

In lieu of such direct examination neuroscientists have been fortunate to be able to turn more and more to technology in their diagnostic and research work. The methods of investigation include X-rays, which provide only indirect knowledge about the brain by means of observations of bone erosion or the displacement or distortion of the fluid-filled ventricles caused by tumor growth or fluid collections. A true representation of the brain itself didn't come until

1972, with the development of X-ray computerized axial tomography (CAT), which was able to distinguish the white matter (composed of nerve fibers and their enclosing myelin sheaths) from the gray matter (made up of the nerve cell bodies). It also provided a means of recognizing alterations in the brain tissue itself. CAT fashions a reconstructed three-dimensional image from a series of two-dimensional projections taken from various angles. Measurements of these X-ray beams are taken by detectors placed in a circular doughnutlike array surrounding the patient's head, and the data resulting from these multiple measurements are reconstructed by computers into a series of images.

The monumental advances provided by procedures like CAT imaging would not have been possible without computers powerful enough to manipulate the immense amount of information generated by these techniques. And since the human brain created the science of computer technology one could even claim that the brain furthered its own evolution and self-understanding by developing technologies capable of overcoming the brain's own limitations. Although I use the word "evolution" somewhat loosely here, I think developments in modern imaging exemplify the truth that the further advancement of our species, particularly in regard to self-understanding, is likely to come from scientific discoveries about our brain's operations rather than from any direct physical modifications in the gross structure of our brains.

The breakthrough in brain imaging made possible by computers soon led to the development of other three-dimensional imaging techniques such as magnetic resonance imaging (MRI). This more sensitive and less hazardous technique (X-rays are not employed) is based on the nuclear energy levels of the nuclei of hydrogen atoms in brain tissue. The nuclei (protons) behave like small magnets when subjected to a strong external magnetic field. If this static magnetic field is perturbed by a radio-frequency pulse of energy, the nuclei are thrown out of alignment and into an increased energy state. When the magnetic field is turned off, the nuclei return to their original state and give off energy in the form of radio-frequency signals that are measured and converted via computer into reconstructed images of high contrast and spatial resolution.

Both CAT and MRI provide structural images of the brain analogous to an architect's blueprint. But neither technique is very informative in terms of measuring the brain's activity. PET scans provide a dynamic picture of brain activity analogous to video, as compared to the still photograph provided by CAT and MRI. PET allows imaging of brain structures along with measurement of the local concentration of injected radioactive tracers. It is based on a very simple principle: those parts of the brain that are most active use up the greatest amount of glucose and require more oxygen than neighboring areas. In this respect the brain is no different from any other organ of the body: All are governed by the laws of thermodynamics, in which energy consumption is directly related to activity. Within seconds of a change in brain activity, local blood flow and metabolism change in tandem. Although the actual changes in neuronal activity occur much faster (a few milliseconds compared to a few hundred milliseconds for blood flow and metabolism) reliable and detailed maps emerge from PET scans of those brain areas involved in a specific activity.

For example, PET makes possible the imaging of the receptors for the brain's ever-expanding list of neurotransmitters. Future refinements are expected to provide detailed chemical maps that show, as does a road map, the points of origin and destination of specific nerve cell pathways. In practical terms such information can provide "pic-

tures" of those parts of the brain involved in normal and disturbed
mental processing. For instance, obsessive-compulsive disorder
(OCD)—traditionally considered a neurosis best treated by psy-
chotherapy—is now recognized as a neuropsychiatric condition
marked by disturbances in three main brain areas: the orbital region
of the frontal cortex, the cingulate cortex just behind, and the head
of the caudate nucleus. On the basis of these findings it's now
thought likely that OCD results from a dysfunction in a orbital
frontal-striatal-thalamic-cortical circuit. Since people with this disorder get better when given drugs that affect levels of the neurotransmitter serotonin, it's likely that a fuller understanding of this
condition (which affects over 2 percent of the population) will come
from additional research on this neurotransmitter and its action
within the circuit.

PET images can also be combined with CAT and MRI images to
provide a composite of brain anatomy and function. For instance,
researchers at the Washington University School of Medicine provided me with three PET images superimposed over an MRI.
Toward the front of the brain an area of activation corresponds to
the subject's thinking about a word; a second area of activation farther back and upward toward the motor area lights up when the subject reads the word; finally, an area at the back of the brain in the
visual area becomes active when the subject just reads the word.

Such studies have already revolutionized our ideas about language
which, it seems, can be broken down into many separate modules
that, acting in concert, are responsible for our species' unique and
highly evolved capacity for language. A similar modular arrangement
is likely for other properties of mind.

PET, CAT, and MRI studies introduced a new era of brain exploration. Still, for all of the insights these techniques have provided,

they have several drawbacks. As noted before, CAT and MRI give information only about structural integrity and say little about the dynamic features of brain activity. While PET is able to capture functional brain activity, the technology is complicated and expensive. The PET device itself costs about a million dollars; the short half-life of the isotopes employed requires the availability of a particle accelerator (cyclotron), at a cost of two to three million dollars; and operation of the system is impossible without a team composed of physicists, radiochemists, nuclear medicine experts, and radiation technologists. Moreover—and this is the greatest shortcoming of all three of these technologies—they do not capture the millisecond intervals in which brain action takes place.

Electroencephalograms (popularly known as "brain wave machines") monitor ongoing electrical activity in the natural temporal duration of brain activity (milliseconds) but supply information principally about electrical signals coming from the surface of the cortex and over too broad a range to be helpful. In addition the signals diffract (bend) as they pass through the skull, producing distortions and resultant confusion as to the signals' origins. Relying on conventional EEGs for specific localizing information is like standing in front of an apartment building and hearing a pistol shot from somewhere inside: you know the gunman is in there *someplace,* but that isn't very helpful in deciding in which apartment to look.

With the aid of computers, high-speed analysis of EEG signals became possible, but unfortunately the gain in speed was offset by differences in interpretation from one human "reader" to another as to the meaning of the peaks, valleys, and plateaus generated on the computer screens. What was needed was a method that provided information that was both localized and closer to "real time," i.e., at the speed information is processed within the brain.

Recently, combined EEG and MRI techniques are meeting both of these goals and shedding light on how thoughts and intentions are formed and translated into commands for action within the brain. Using a model that integrates MRI information with 128-electrode EEG recordings, neuroscientists at the EEG Systems Laboratory in San Francisco challenged airline pilots to sit in front of a computer screen and watch a stream of numbers. They were asked to hold in mind two numbers while the screen went blank for a few seconds. When a third number then appeared on the screen the pilots had to push a pressure-sensitive button with a force proportional to the first number in the sequence seen some twelve seconds earlier.

Prior to the appearance of the target number many brain areas come into play corresponding to activated circuits in the premotor and left posterior parietal cortex. The color-coded images of this enhanced cortical activity resemble the bolts of lightning that appeared in comic strips of the fifties and sixties.

In fact, Dr. Allen Givens, the developer of the combined technique, speaks of these colorful bolts as shadows of thought—early indicators that the brain was shaping and anticipating its responses according to the demands of the experiment.

Support for this interpretation came when the experiment was repeated with the test subjects again requested to press the pressure-sensitive button, but this time with the opposite hand. A different anticipatory pattern emerged, implying different circuits employed according to different conditions and strategies of response.

Another neuroimaging technique relies on measurements of the tiny magnetic fields created by neurons. When activated, the neurons create an electric current that induces a magnetic field measurable by the SQUID device (an acronym for superconducting quantum interference device). The SQUID sensors record magnetic flux. The principal advantage of magnetoencephalography (MEG) is its higher shutter speed. While PET can only take "snapshots" of the brain separated by anywhere from a quarter of a second to ten seconds, and MRI requires at least a full second, MEG measurements capture brain action in real time with temporal resolution in the range of tens of milliseconds.

Within one hundred milliseconds after an individual sees something his speech areas light up, a first reflection of the intention to speak. In another experiment carried out at New York University volunteers closed their eyes and tried to come up with a word that rhymed with a test word. As they did so suppression of the normal alpha activity occurred over the visual cortex for more than five hundred milliseconds, followed, one hundred milliseconds later, by suppression over the speech area in the lateral temporal regions—a pattern reflecting the brain's first visualizing the word and then activating its memory and speech areas to come up with a word with a similar sound. Other counterintuitive findings from SQUID studies reveal that red and green stimuli provoke responses in different parts of the visual cortex and loud sounds are processed in different brain areas from quieter sounds.

One final technique, functional magnetic resonance imaging (fMRI), first demonstrated in 1991, is a souped-up version of the conventional MRI. It makes possible the recording of "movies" of the brain as it thinks, remembers, experiences emotions, and even dreams. It works by measuring a faint difference in the magnetic signal between fully oxygenated blood taken up by the active nerve cells, and the deoxygenated blood resulting from the extraction of oxygen by those nerve cells. The fast MRI pinpoints these faint signals and, via computer enhancement, creates movies of the activated brain. Early research supports PET and MEG results showing that multiple and often widely separated brain areas may be involved in mental processing. Indeed the technologies are bringing about a profound modification in our ideas about how the brain works.

Recall the theory of John Hughlings Jackson, who held that the brain is organized hierarchically. Until the development of fMRI, neuroscientists could only speculate about whether Jackson's theory was correct. Now they have their proof. In 1993 a team from the University of Wisconsin used an fMRI to study what happens in the brain as volunteers undertook increasingly complicated motor tasks. They found that simple movement of a finger activated the primary motor cortex on the opposite side of the body. If a more complex movement was called for (touching each finger to the thumb in rapid succession), additional brain areas came into play, including the nearby supplementary motor area (SMA), the sensory cortex on the opposite side, and the premotor cortex on both sides.

The SMA findings are particularly revealing since that area is considered a higher order "supramotor" center involved in the programming and production of complex movements. It was never active in simple movements but only in complex ones; in addition, it became selectively active even when the subjects were requested to merely *imagine* carrying out a complex movement. Thus a hierarchy for movement exists within the brain, starting with the SMA and premotor cortex, which plan and integrate the intended movement, followed by the engagement of the motor and sensory cortex at the moment the movement is carried out. And as discussed earlier, the sequence may be started prior to conscious awareness and thus call into question who or what is initiating it. Further additional activity in other brain areas cannot be excluded as a contributing factor, though, because even fMRI may not be sensitive enough to detect it.

As a result of such studies, unthinkable prior to the development of fMRI, concepts like "mind," "will," and "imagination" are taking on neurologic significance. Moving objects through space in one's imagination activates nearby but nonetheless different brain areas than those used in actually moving the object. And certain personalities are turning out to exhibit distinct fMRI patterns. For instance, different areas of the brain are activated in obsessive compulsives than in normal subjects when each encounters a dreaded situation he or she is trying to avoid. In the near future neuroscientists will be able to diagnose and formulate treatments for brain diseases, as well as make educated guesses about personality and "cognitive style" (how a person uses memory, his patterns of thinking and response) on the bases of "brainprints" composed of a combination of MRI, PET, MEG, fMRI, and who knows what other emerging technologies. Moreover, radioactive tags will be put on the brain's neurotransmitters, as well as on any drug that can be employed to influence the brain, to provide "snapshots" of the chemistry underlying brain activity.

Despite these advances, I believe certain conceptual barriers will continue to frustrate our attempts at completely correlating the world of inner mental experience with neuroimaging. In my book *The Brain* (1984), I described a situation that at the time was pure science fiction, but that since then has become possible. Let me present it again in briefer form:

Imagine yourself as an neuroradiologist sitting with a colleague and looking at a PET scan. As you examine the image you notice activity in the occipital region, containing the visual areas, toward the back of the brain. "Looks like the subject is being visually stimulated," you mention to your colleague. As you do so the PET pattern changes to show activity toward the front in the prefrontal areas, which are important in planning, as well as in the left hemisphere, principally the speech area. At this point, if you are astute enough, you have all of the information required to make a tentative guess that you are, in fact, looking at a PET scan of your own brain. Prior to the moment you formulate this hypothesis, the situation concerned one brain, yours, studying the brain of an unknown subject. How did that situation change with your realization that by some means or other you are studying the moment-to-moment operation of your own brain? For one thing, you now are aware of the neurologic correlates of your own mental operations, watching areas of your brain change from moment to moment, a form of self-knowledge previously unavailable to you. As another way of putting it, your brain is studying itself via the PET scan. But since you feel in control in this situation—you can alter the PET scan in various ways by deliberate acts such as, say, turning on the stereo in the viewing room and thus activating the music appreciation center in the right hemisphere—you feel that your *mind* is directing the operations of your brain. But as a brain specialist you are uncomfortable with this hypothesis, since your knowledge of the brain has led you to the belief that the mind is best defined as the operation of the brain.

A better, counterintuitive way of thinking about this situation is to consider that consciousness—your self-awareness that you are looking at your own PET scan—was merely the activation of an additional brain activity: a consciousness module, so to speak. While this explanation sounds reasonable enough, it isn't completely convincing. Consciousness is a subjective experience that is qualitatively different from the actions of looking, talking, and listening done earlier. What's more, we accord to our own consciousness a privileged defining position and identify completely with it. Our individual consciousness cannot be experienced by anyone other than ourselves, nor can it be located in the brain by PET or any other device.

A gap exists between the world of inner experience and its demonstration by any neuroimaging device now available or foreseeable in the near future. That's because the inner subjective world of our own inner experience exists separate from any technological demonstration of brain activity. We can always change our "mind" or alter our strategy for the most whimsical reasons. No neuroimaging device can portray our capacities for unpredictability, arbitrariness, even just plain irascible uncooperativeness. That is the wonder and the power of human freedom.

One of the unsolved mysteries of the human brain raised by the new technology is described by Rodolfo Llinas, Professor of Neuroscience at New York University: "How are the separate bits of activity in different parts of the brain made into a single event?" As an example, consider my present situation: while I am typing these words I am also dimly aware of the traffic passing outside the window in front of me, the sound of Mozart playing in the background, and the feeling of being slightly chilled in the early morning grayness. While each of these sensations is occurring separately I experience them as components of an integrated whole. Somehow each of these sensations is bound together within the brain into one integrated experience. But how? A common sense explanation would hold that at some as yet undetermined area of the brain all of the various components of experience are synthesized into a unity. But so far neuroscientists haven't discovered such a Master Control Center, leading many of them to conclude that the brain must employ other means to synthesize the separate components of our mental life into a unity.

One influential theory holds that the binding is not a spatial but a temporal one. According to Dr. Llinas, a 40-cycle-per-second wave sweeps the brain from front to back every 12.5-thousandth of a second. He believes this wave serves to link information from those parts of the cortex handling vision, hearing, and other sensations, with the *thalamus,* the lower brain structure that is a way station for sensory impulses on their way to the cerebral cortex. One of the nuclei of the thalamus, the *intralaminar* nucleus, is particularly suited to carry out such a temporal integration. It sends out axons to almost every part of the cortex and acts as a reception center for returning axons from these same areas. Thus the thalamus and cortex are intimately connected. And since the intralaminar nucleus fires at a 40 cycle per second rate, Dr. Llinas believes this firing rhythm is the source of that same rhythmicity he measures at the cortical surface. According to Llinas's theory the integration of something like my writing experience mentioned above depends on the interaction between the scanning wave originating in the thalamus and the active sensory cells in the cortex. Every 12.5-thousandth of a second the thalamus's intralaminar nucleus sends out its wave, which influences the active cells in the sensory cortex to entrain to the same frequency as the intralaminar cells (40 cycles per second) and send back to the thalamus a train of nervous impulses precisely timed to the 40-cycles-per-second rhythm. Thus the sensory components of traffic sounds, Mozart, and the early morning chill are experienced as a unity rather than three separate components. So far, though, no one has come up with an explanation for why a 40 Hz wave and no other should enjoy such a privileged status.

And this is just one of the many uncertainties about the brain's principles of operation. One of the reasons that it remains so mysterious is that it is governed by both mechanical and quantum principles. As a result the brain is inherently indeterminant, unpredictable, and uncertain. For instance, at the cellular level the "firing" of a neuron is dependent on the ratio of excitatory influences (via excitatory neurotransmitters) to inhibitory ones (via inhibitory neurotransmitters). At the molecular layer this translates into whether or not a synaptic vesicle will discharge its contents into the synaptic space. But this action cannot be predicted, since synaptic vesicles are so small they are governed by quantum rules and are inherently indeterminate. Thus we can only speak of the "probability" that the vesicle will discharge its contents—no one can predict for certain—which does away with the possibility of predicting brain activity on the molecular scale. The same holds true, of course, on the macromolecular scale of the whole brain and the whole organism. The plethora of psychological theories—not one of which can offer more than a probability estimate of how a particular human being will respond from one moment to the next—mirrors on the larger scale of human behavior the quantum indeterminism of the brain.

Despite the emphasis on the individual cell and its connections in the above description, neurons do not act alone but as components of networks. What's more, these networks interact in dynamic patterns that change according to circumstances. We know this as a result of experiments in which limb movements have been correlated with those areas of the brain responsible for the movement. Since these experiments involve opening the skull and inserting electrodes into the brains of perfectly normal creatures, it should come as no surprise to learn that monkeys rather than humans have been the experimental subjects. Considerable variation exists from one monkey to another in regard to the locations at which the electrical shock induced movement in the monkey's hand. Moreover, the "map" relating brain area to hand movement changes over time. Just as the borders of a country change to reflect natural and human-produced changes, the brain alters itself on the basis of experience. In the monkey experiment the "brain map" was altered by the cruel act of cutting off one of the monkey's fingers. Within the next several weeks the neurons formerly controlling that finger were incorporated into the brain areas representing one or more of the remaining fingers. This was not guided by genetic "instructions" but was a manifestation of the brain's dynamic power to organize itself in response to changing circumstances by altering the connectivity patterns of neurons. In essence, the brain consists of ever-changing networks of relationships. This means that information is not localized into neat pigeonholes but is distributed throughout its 50 billion neurons.

A study of braille reading among the blind provides another example of brain modification through experience. Researchers discovered that a larger amount of the cortex is assigned to the finger used by the subjects for reading—the right index finger—than for the left index finger of the same subjects; the amount of cortex is also larger than that that assigned to either the right or left index finger of individuals with normal vision. In this case, a change in behavior—the learning and practice of reading braille—led to a remodeling of the sensory representations of the involved body part: the brain refashioned itself to enhance the importance of the finger involved in braille reading.

According to Gerald M. Edelman, Nobel laureate and director of the Neurosciences Institute at The Scripps Research Institute, additional complexity within the brain comes from the action of neurons that are not directly affected by the external world but "talk" only to one another. While many nerve cells link us to the outside world by mediating sensation and movement, the majority of neurons communicate only with other neurons. Indeed, the brain is more in touch with itself than with anything else. This makes for several unique features.

For one thing, the brain literally creates itself during our earliest development. At various times in the developmental process from fetus to newborn to infant, nerve cells migrate, many die off, and many others stick to one another and send out processes whereby neuronal connections are formed and re-formed. This orchestration depends upon sensitivities on the part of the developing brain to *place* (the effect of other cells in the immediate area), *time* (the brain develops in designated stages, and if development is thwarted the brain often cannot later compensate), and the chemical and electrical *activity* of neighboring neurons.

In a theory of brain development he calls neuronal group selection, Edelman proposes that environmental experiences throughout our lifetime influence the creation of neuronal circuits. Only those circuits that are helpful in adapting us to our environment are created and preserved. Other cell connections that are not helpful in adaptation are not preserved—accounting for the enormous number of nerve cells that disappear early in brain development and, to a lesser extent, throughout our life span. As a result of this process of neuronal group selection, brains evolve within a given species that, to superficial observation, look very much alike but at the microscopic level—the network of nerve cell connections among billions of cells—differ enormously. This variation extends even to identical twins, since no two people ever experience the same things in exactly the same way.

How does one describe so dynamic a process, which occurs over time scales extending from milliseconds to the seven or eight decades of the human life span? In *Bright Air, Brilliant Fire*, Edelman suggests an analogy:

"The chemical and electrical dynamics of the brain resemble the sound and light patterns and the movement and growth patterns of a jungle. . . . Indeed the circuits of the brain look like no others. The neurons have treelike arbors that overlap and ramify in myriad ways.

Their signaling is . . . like the vast aggregate of interactive events in a jungle."

Within a jungle nothing is stable from moment to moment; so, too, in the brain. Even as I write these words and you read them, our brains are altered by new information that brings about multi-layered structural changes:

". . . [B]rain development, brain action, and mental activity . . . involve vast numbers of cells with electrical activity and chemical diversity, an enormously intricate anatomy with blobs and sheets linked in rich ways, and maps that receive signals from sensory input and send signals to motor output. These structures undergo continuous electrical and chemical change. . . ."

The changes within the brain necessary for its development come about through the evolutionary mechanism of natural selection: "From genes to proteins, from cells to orderly development, from electrical activity to neurotransmitter release, from sensory sheets to maps, from shape to function and behavior, from social communication back to any and all of these levels, we are confronted with a system . . . that is continually subjected to natural selection."

From these multilevel interactions whereby some nerve cell circuits are enhanced while others disappear altogether emerges the mind and all of its properties. And events at one level can affect all others. A slight variation in the genes and an aberrant chemical may alter brain development so as to produce a retarded or mentally ill person. Less devastating alterations within the genetic or chemical makeup of the brain may result in subtle personality changes, perhaps a tendency toward shyness or introversion accompanied by attendant problems in self-esteem. Or the process can work from the top down, as when the *mind* of a martyr or a saint chooses death, the destruction of brain and mind rather than renunciation of a cherished belief.

Moreover, these multilevel interactions extend over a lifetime, reflecting the individual's perceptions, activities, and habits. Even in old age the brain continues to undergo changes dependent on the richness, novelty, and challenges that one encounters or sets for oneself. We essentially create our own brains by means of the choices that we make about how we will live our lives. Based on each person's unique life experiences, certain connections among neurons are strengthened or weakened with the aid of specific biochemical processes. Thus functioning circuits are selectively "carved out" within the brain's vast assemblage of billions of neurons, and interact and mutually influence one another.

As an example, the visual system of the monkey contains over twenty different maps for such things as orientation, color, and movement. (A similar arrangement is considered highly likely in the human brain as well.) Correlation and coordination of these different processes occur by mutual interaction. In this way the connections between neurons within certain groups are strengthened, while others are weakened or disappear altogether. Because all such networking takes place absent a "supervisor" to summarize or correlate the information flowing within these different maps, it is impossible to predict the outcome of the activity of large numbers of mutually interacting neurons. This is another example of the brain's inherent unpredictability: It allows only rough statistical correlations between brain function and mental processes. Moreover, inherent limitations exist that limit the brain's ability to intuit, through conscious awareness, the principles of its own operation. We know this as a result of what has been learned about the specialized functions of the two cerebral hemispheres.

The corpus callosum, the largest bundle of nerve fibers in the brain (the term means "thick-skinned body"), transfers information along its 800 million connections from one hemisphere to the other. Because of its size and midline position, this structure has always seemed a promising avenue of research into the unity of consciousness. One psychologist even tried persuading a neurosurgeon to promise that, in the event the psychologist should ever contract a fatal illness, the neurosurgeon would cut the psychologist's corpus callosum so that he could personally investigate any changes in his own conscious awareness!

A less bizarre approach to testing this hunch—the neurosurgeon sensibly demurred—came in the early 1970s, when Roger Sperry and several of his graduate students evaluated several epileptic patients who had undergone a surgical splitting of their corpora callosa. The operation was based on a sound but rather radical approach to seizure control: with the corpus callosum divided, seizure discharges could no longer travel from their point of origin in one hemisphere across the corpus to their opposite neighbor. Sperry found that, in the words of Jerre Levy, one of his graduate students, "each side of the brain was a fully human organ of thought, each specialized for a set of functions that were complementary to that of the opposite hemisphere."

To summarize a great deal of research: Things are perceived and analyzed as a whole by the right hemisphere, whereas the left hemisphere breaks things down into their components. The right hemisphere excels at reading maps, working out jigsaw puzzles, copying designs, distinguishing and remembering musical tones, recognizing faces, analyzing other people's emotions via the interpretation of their tones of voice or facial expression (essentially the reading of "body language"), visualizing in three-dimensional space, and other activities involving perceptual-spatial relations. In addition to language, the left hemisphere is involved in all other activities that involve analysis or sequential processing.

The hemisphere that is activated in a given situation also depends on the nature of the particular task being attempted. For instance, since the right hemisphere does better with facial recognition most people are better at identifying a familiar picture among a group of pictures if all of the pictures are displayed in the left visual field. (Remember: Each side of the brain controls the opposite side of the body.) But if the facial pictures are turned upside down, it doesn't matter in which visual field the pictures are placed. Context matters.

Another example of context, an unexpected and seemingly magical one when first observed, involves the response of a split-brain patient to a special picture known as a chimeric figure. One of my favorite chimeric figures was made by cutting in half a photograph of the actress Catherine Deneuve and combining one half of it with half of a second picture taken of a dockworker in San Francisco.

After being joined together at the midline, this strange hybrid is then flashed rapidly on a screen in such a way that the half showing the actress goes to the right hemisphere and the other half depicting the dockworker goes to the left. The split-brain subject's identification of what she has just seen depends on the method employed to elicit the information. If the examiner asks, "What did you just see?" she answers, "A suntanned, burly man." But if she is asked to point to what she saw she selects from an array the whole picture of Catherine Deneuve. These differing responses result from selective activation of the two hemispheres. The direct question asked by the examiner activated the language hemisphere on the left, which then provided a verbal description of what it saw. The request to point toward what was seen did not involve language but visual spatial orientation, mediated by the right hemisphere. The subject then pointed to the actress's half-picture, since that was the one perceived by that hemisphere.

Such experiments underscore the fact that the two hemispheres, when operating separately, go about structuring "reality" in different ways. Moreover, each hemisphere's special processing operations lend a richness to perception and behavior. In split-brain patients this specialization of the hemispheres is exaggerated, since each operates in isolation from the other. For the rest of us, the two hemispheres share the fruits of their separate operations: we do not perceive different worlds but a single, unified one from different aspects. (It should be added that even the split-brain patient doesn't experience two separate worlds, since he is consciously aware of only those mediated by the left hemisphere.) This is because the corpus callosum enables each hemisphere to communicate to the other its unique ordering and processing of the world.

To get a clearer sense of the specific activities of the two hemispheres, imagine yourself at a lecture. The speaker's words are analyzed by your left hemisphere, while the speaker's general "manner" (i.e., his tone of voice, his enthusiasm or lack of it, his overall "likability" and "credibility") is interpreted by your right hemisphere. Most likely these right-brain perceptions rise no higher in your consciousness than a vague "intuition." If asked to explain why you like or dislike the speaker, you may grope for words and concepts to bolster that intuition. Perhaps the lecturer used the word "brilliant" to describe one of the questions put to him by a member of the audience, yet his pronunciation of that word conveyed sarcasm, as if he really thought the question rather stupid.

An impairment in the right hemisphere deprives a person of the ability to make such determinations based on another person's general manner. This occurs because the left hemisphere can deal only with the actual meaning of the words and must leave emotional nuances to its right-hemisphere compatriot. Similarly, a person with damage to the right hemisphere also has difficulty with the production of emotional speech, such as sounding sarcastic on demand. (In a psychological experiment testing this ability he may be asked to "pretend" certain emotions.) As a result of such receptive and expressive failures the person with right-hemisphere damage sounds "flat" and "robotic."

Why would the human brain have evolved in such a way that the two hemispheres process information in different ways? And which hemisphere best captures what is "really" going on in the world? The only true answer is that each hemisphere encodes different aspects of the world according to its own specialized manner and communicates that information to its partner. At every moment in the normal brain, the two hemispheres are receiving the same stimulus but extracting different information from it. Each hemisphere is processing not only its own sensory information at all times, but also the results of the other hemisphere's processing of the same information (i.e., in terms of the above example: while the left hemisphere works on the meanings of words in a sentence, it is receiving and incorporating perceptions from the right hemisphere concerning "tone" of voice). As to the advantage of such an arrangement neuropsychologist Jerre Levy suggests:

"In collaboration, operating on the same information from the same world of real-life experiences, the two hemispheres are able to build up representations that are far more complete, veridical, and rich in information than would be possible for either hemisphere alone or for two hemispheres that were functional clones. By virtue of the enormous information-carrying capacity of the corpus callosum, the power and generality of these mental models extend over the whole domain of experience, not just the portion that is the province of one or the other hemisphere."

In short, neither hemisphere provides a "truer" version of reality but, rather, different though complementary aspects of it. Dualism is thus wired into our very biology. A few pages back we spoke of dualisms such as holism versus localization and the neuron versus the nerve net theory. Such dichotomies, in which both sides of the controversy are true in some respects and neither ever quite vanquishes the other, should not be surprising in light of what we now know about the distinctive operations of the two hemispheres of our brain. The brain has evolved into an inherently dialectic organ that attempts during every moment of its existence to achieve a unification of opposites. Thought and emotion, art and science, yin and yang, the literal and the metaphorical, the true and the illusory—these are only some of the dualisms that this inherently dualistic organ wrestles with. And the advantage of such an arrangement? One hemisphere acts as a corrective for the other. Both the words *and* the underlying tone of voice are necessary in order to arrive at the meaning of a particular utterance.

One or other of the hemisphere's operations can be favored at different times and under certain conditions. In a courtroom the jury is instructed to decide strictly on the basis of logic, as developed via verbal reasoning, the determination of whether one side has made its "case." Reliance on intuition or on such things as reading the "body language" of the various participants is forbidden—an injunction that if adhered to effectively eliminates the contributions of the right hemisphere. ("Surprise" verdicts may actually result from the jury's intentional or unintentional reliance on the "gut reactions" mediated by the right hemisphere.) In the arts the situation is often just the opposite. Appreciation of abstractionist or nonrepresentational art demands that language and logic yield place to the perception of pure form, color, and other right-hemisphere-mediated qualities.

Emerging knowledge of the organization and functioning of the two hemispheres led in the 1970s to the oversimplified notion that people can be divided into "right" and "left" brain types, and courses of instruction in painting and writing soon began to encourage students to develop their "right brain." Such teachings ignored the fact that, except under the rare and unnatural conditions of a split-brain operation, we possess two integrated hemispheres that are in constant two-way communication with each other across the corpus callosum. And although it is true that some people's thought patterns and behavior seem more expressive of one hemisphere than the other (lawyer, left, versus potter, right), this does not imply that such individuals are not using both brain hemispheres. The lawyer may spend his leisure time attending or listening to operas while the potter must have some rudimentary understanding of commerce if he is ever to succeed in getting others to purchase his work. In short, we possess a *unified* brain.

In my book *The Modular Brain* (1994) I developed in considerable detail a few of the fascinating and intellectually intriguing philosophical consequences issuing from our newfound knowledge about the two hemispheres. Let me describe here only one of many similar experiments that raise important questions about the integration of the human personality.

When J. W., a split-brain patient of neurolopsychologist Michael Gazzaniga, is shown for less than a second a picture of a horse flashed only to his right hemisphere, he denies that he has seen anything. But when asked to draw "what goes on it," he picks up a pencil with his left hand and draws an English saddle, a rather primitive drawing difficult to interpret outside of the context of the experiment. The patient doesn't recognize what he has drawn. He is then asked to draw, rather than say, what picture has been flashed. With his left hand he then draws a horse and, after completing the picture, he grins and says of the first drawing: "That must be a saddle."

Was J.W. aware that he had just seen a horse? The answer is both yes and no. If we emphasize what he says, we would have to conclude an absence of awareness. Yet if we emphasize J.W.'s behavior, the correctness of his responses clearly indicates knowledge. Moreover, he not only knows, albeit at a subverbal level, what he has just seen, he can also reason about it and make inferences—all done prior to his becoming consciously aware of the horse by means of his second drawing. This disparity between reported experience and behavior raises difficulties only if we persist in granting more importance to what people *say* about their experience than to what they do. Yet behavior rather than self-reporting of subjective, internal events is a more reliable indicator of a person's intentions. ("Actions speak louder than words.") From the neurobiologic point of view, too, this principle makes a good deal of sense, since the brain evolved in order to make increasingly sophisticated responses to an increasingly complicated environment. The frontal lobes, those brain areas associated most closely with the higher expressions of the human mind, are contiguous with the motor tracts, which em*body* our intentions via specific actions. But what of the freedom of our actions? Are we constrained by circumstances, specifically the circumstances of our own brain's organization?

With that last question we encounter one of the most contentious controversies about human behavior. While we inwardly experience ourselves from moment to moment as free to think and act as we will, a respectable number of philosophers in the past have claimed that our inner conviction of freedom is illusory. Supporting this view are certain insights gained from psychiatry and "abnormal psychology" (more correctly, the psychology of the "abnormal" mind).

Most notable in this regard are the results of research on obsessions and compulsions: intrusive, unwanted, even reprehensible thoughts, and repetitive, ritualized behaviors. A person suffering from obsessive-compulsive disorder (OCD), may, for instance, experience a gnawing, irrepressible sense of being contaminated. He recognizes such a thought as irrational but cannot help thinking it; nor can he stop the washing and cleansing rituals that, however often and diligently performed, fail in their purpose of ridding himself of these irrational thoughts and behavioral patterns.

Traditional explanations of OCD concentrated on psychological explanations, derived mainly from psychoanalysis. (Fixation or regression on the part of the patient to the "anal" stage of psychosexual development was one favorite.) But hints have long existed suggesting an alternative explanation for OCD. For instance, brain inflammation was a major symptom in the 1919 worldwide epidemic of influenza. Many of the patients so affected developed movement disorders such as uncontrollable tics and repetitive motions. Accompanying these motor disturbances were behaviors typical of obsessive compulsives, such as those described by a psychiatrist of his postencephalitic patient:

"He worried over disturbing ideas, whether his employer or his employer's wife was insulted by certain things he might have said, whether he really had closed the window, whether the door of the room was properly closed. He would wash his hands repeatedly during these episodes, look under the bed to see if anyone were hiding there, and dust his chair carefully before seating himself."

Soon other brain diseases were discovered to be associated with OCD. An early clue to the anatomical circuitry involved in the illness came from the success of a drastic treatment for the disorder that involved cutting the nerve fibers from the frontal cortex to subcortical sites such as the basal ganglia. This observation was eventually correlated with a no less puzzling illness that struck a French noblewoman.

In 1825, neurologist Jean Itard reported on the Marquise de Dampierre, who developed persistent symptoms of bodily tics, barking like a dog, and the uttering of uncontrollable obscenities. So disturbing were these symptoms to herself and others that the Marquise lived as a recluse until her death in her eighties. Over sixty years later neurologist Georges Gilles de la Tourette wrote of the marquise and eight other people with multiple tics, involuntary movements, and the tendency to shout obscenities (coprolalia) and to echo back the spoken words of others (echolalia). Tourette believed the symptoms of the disorder occurred involuntarily, and thus exactly opposite of the way that obsessive-compulsive disorders were thought to happen. For this reason the two disorders were "adopted" by different specialists of the human mind: OCD was appropriated by the psychiatrists who remained convinced of its psychological origins and spun elaborate theories to account for it; Tourette's remained under the banner of the neurologists who emphasized the motor tics and inquired little about their patients' inner experiences. During my own training years I don't recall any reference to OCD by my neurology professors, nor anything said about Tourette's by my psychiatric instructors.

In 1980 all of this changed as the result of an extraordinary essay that appeared in the *Archives of General Psychiatry*. The writer, a patient, identified as Joseph Bliss, described his observations of his own Tourette's:

"I have been stalking this thing for over 35 years with a single-minded determination to find something that would give me a clue, a direction, to the meaning of the problem."

He found that "faint signals" preceded his unusual movements. He described them as "vague unfulfilled feelings," which merged into "discrete sensations."

"Each movement is preceded by certain preliminary sensory signals" and is the result of "a voluntary capitulation to a demanding and relentless urge accompanied by an extraordinarily subtle sensation that provokes and fuels the urge. Successively sharper movements build up to a climax, a climax that never comes. . . . The Tourette's syndrome movements are intentional bodily movements. The intention is to relieve a sensation, as surely as the movement to scratch an itch is to relieve the itch. If the itch was so subtle and fast that it escaped detection, would that make the act any less voluntary?"

Bliss's emphasis on the voluntariness of the movements flew in the face of every expert on the illness since Tourette himself, for it was precisely the involuntariness of the movements, the patient's inability to control them, that formed the hallmark of the condition.

Thirteen years later Bliss's claims were put to the test and compared to the experiences of 135 people with the disorder. Ninety-three percent reported "premonitory urges"; a similar percentage reported that their tics were either fully or partially a voluntary response to the premonitory urges and accompanied by a feeling of relief.

Such findings blurred the margins between Tourette's and obsessive-compulsive disorder, which is marked by a conscious—indeed, hyperconscious—awareness accompanying an internal demand to think a certain thought (obsession) or perform a certain act (compulsion). Indeed, some patients coming to the attention of psychiatrists or neurologists defied any exact classification under a single disorder.

Typical in this respect is Carey, a patient of mine who began at an early age to make barking noises, grunt, and frequently clear his throat. He also exhibited jerking movements of his head and neck along with twitches of the face. Taking only these behaviors into account, Carey would be accurately described as suffering from Tourette's. But careful inquiry revealed that this patient also led a hidden psychological life constructed around a series of rituals concerning numbers. He did everything possible to avoid encountering the numbers 6 or 3. For instance, he always turned off his television on channel 32 or any other number whose digits would not add up to 3 or 6 or a multiple of them. He couldn't get into bed until the hour and minute hand added up to a "safe" number. When drinking a glass of water he silently counted so as to put the glass down on 5 or 7 but never 6. When his girlfriend once told him she loved him he replied in kind, and then became uncomfortable when she repeated her declaration another time, bringing the total to 3. He then said it again to end the number of "I love you"s on 4. When closing a window he found he had to check it and touch it seven times. Finally, Carey had difficulty stopping himself from asking other people a series of questions in invariant order, questions usually concerning their previous whereabouts. If they didn't answer in a set manner he had to ask the questions again in exactly the same sequence. Friends, and eventually his girlfriend, broke off with Carey because of their unwillingness to undergo what they considered senseless and intrusive interrogations.

Does Carey suffer from two illnesses—Tourette's and OCD—or only one? Here is what Carey himself has concluded: "I can control these rituals to some extent, at least I can delay them or force myself by tremendous effort to ignore 3s and 6s. But with the noises and the movements I have no control, because my body seems to be doing it despite me. Sometimes I will be making a noise or a movement and don't even know that I'm doing it. It's as if my will is involved with the rituals and I can maintain some limited control whereas the movements and the sounds come from my body and not my mind."

Although he doesn't know it, Carey is a modern-day Cartesian: an advocate of Descartes's opinion that the mind can be considered apart from the body. But as I trust I have convinced you by now, such distinctions are fraught with peril from both the logical and the neurologic point of view.

PET studies of OCD show three areas of abnormally high activity: the orbital portion of the frontal cortex, the cingulate cortex (an area about midway between the front and back of the cerebral hemispheres), and the head of the caudate nucleus. The caudate is, of course, one component of the basal ganglia—the area thought to have been affected in the 1919 influenza epidemic. As another indication of their importance in obsession and compulsion, surgically cutting the fibers projecting from the orbital cortex to the basal ganglia or, as an alternative, severing the cingulate, can eliminate or at least vastly improve the symptoms.

Neuroscientists now regard OCD as the result of some abnormality along a circuit that includes the frontal cortex, the basal ganglia, the thalamus, and the cingulate cortex. Thus Carey's distinction between the "mind and will" versus the "body" may represent the subjective experiencing of different points of origin of the disturbance within this circuit.

"One might speculate that in the subjects with obsessive-compulsive disorder and Tourette's syndrome, the compulsion arises de novo, or before a conscious thought, and thus arises from a subcortical trigger, possibly from the basal ganglia or thalamus. For the subjects with obsessive-compulsive disorder in which it is known that there is orbital-frontal hyperactivity, the stimulus starts as a thought arising from the frontal lobe, which then triggers a compulsion," says Mark S. George, a psychiatrist at the National Institutes of Mental Health.

Most likely, Tourette's and OCD represent different outer expressions (phenotypes, as the biologists refer to them) of the same underlying disorder stemming from a dysfunction that emanates from the same underlying gene. While most affected individuals fall under the classification of one or the other of the two illnesses, a smaller percentage are like Carey who suffers from, as he characterizes it, disorders of both the mind and the body.

Carey's illness provides an important insight into the relationship of the mental and the physical. What separates the two is not some form of material, physical existence versus nonmaterial existence (however that may be explained), but, instead, the degree of conscious awareness involved. When Carey makes sounds he is often completely unaware (i.e., unconscious) that he is doing so. But his OCD experiences occur in what seems to him a heightened state of consciousness in which, it appears, he can think of nothing else. These seemingly different experiences result from activation at different sites in a circuit. Activation further forward and upward (the frontal cortex) produces hyperawareness, while activation below the cortex in the basal ganglia induces automatic activity that occurs out-side of conscious awareness and control.

Experience with patients like Carey suggests to me that our future understanding of topics like "consciousness" and "awareness" will emerge not from traditional philosophy and psychology but from the brain sciences. Moreover it is likely that new findings about the brain will force us to revise our ideas about some of the mental capacities we pretty much take for granted. In England a group of subjects known in the literature as the "K" family provides an example.

Members of the "K" family suffer from a most unusual disorder. Although they are all of at least normal intelligence and exhibit no obvious behavioral or social maladjustments, they cannot seem to speak normally. Even apparently simple sentences come out sound-ing odd and disjointed. They speak ungrammatically and have difficulty with tenses and pronouns. Typical of their difficulties is a sentence like "I walking down the road."

Known as specific language impairment (SLI) or developmental dyslexia, this strange disorder is inherited by as yet incompletely understood mechanisms. It affects identical twins (who share the same genes) much more often than fraternal twins (who share only about half their genes). When the disturbance runs in a family it affects about one in four individuals.

MRI scans of individuals with SLI reveal an enlargement of the right perisylvian area—an area of brain tissue known to be involved in language processing. This abnormality is thought to impose an inherited biological risk for language difficulties. What's needed to convert that risk into the full-blown syndrome is an elevation in testosterone levels during early brain development.

SLI is of interest because most people, including most neurosci-entists, don't usually think of an ability like using correct grammar as having a specific locus within the brain. We intend to say certain things in our native language and we . . . just say them. But SLI suggests that things are not quite so simple. Even something as effortless as the speaking of simple sentences depends upon the integrity of grammatical circuits within the brain. Recent research has even revealed that different brain areas are involved in the processing of regular verbs ("talk" and "talked") and irregular verbs ("sweep" and "swept").

Other research indicates that a person's ability to estimate size ("Which is bigger, an ant or an elephant?") can disappear under electrical stimulation of a particular brain area in the left hemisphere. Thus, not only our language but, it seems, most aspects of our thinking (some linguists would claim *all* of our thinking) depend upon brain organization and functioning. A slipup at the level of gross anatomy (an abnormality of one of the main structural components), or at the level of the neuron or connections within a circuit, and our most treasured mental capacities may be impaired.

V

Over the next decade new and innovative ways of understanding normal personality are likely to emerge. Up to now most theories on the subject have relied heavily on concepts drawn from the psychiatrist's consulting room. The "introvert," for instance, is regarded as only an attenuated version of the total self-absorption of the psychotic; the "extrovert" as a less exaggerated form of the manic. But the normal personality cannot be understood as simply a kind of watered-down version of the extremes of the neurotic or the psychotic. It exists on its own terms and is best understood without reference to mental illnesses. Temperament, for instance, is a dynamic trait built upon genetics, environment, and life experience. Identifying and describing these interrelated influences over the centuries have commanded the talents of both scientists and artists.

While Hippocrates' explanation of a personality based on humors had more art than science about it, a contemporary theory espoused by psychiatrist and geneticist Robert Cloninger intermixes the sciences of genetics, neuroscience, and mathematics. He posits four basic components of personality: reward dependence, harm avoidance, novelty seeking, and persistence. A person who seeks only the avoidance of pain and discomfort is likely to settle for less in life than the novelty seeker, who views such an orientation as an intolerable bore and emphasizes that life involves risks and unpredictable though always exciting changes in fortune.

Cloninger's four-dimensional grid makes it possible to predict not only how a person may feel about and react to a particular situation but even whether he or she is likely to react to a particular drug. For instance, Cloninger found that people who rate high in harm avoidance and reward dependence (traits that put them at the passive, socially dependent end of the social continuum) respond favorably to medications like Prozac.

Subsequent refinements are likely to link personality, character, and neurotransmitter profiles that more accurately reflect brain chemistry. These new and more comprehensive explanations are likely to include a person's reaction to chemical substances. For instance, a favorable response to drugs activating the dopamine system is one current way of identifying people suffering from forms of attention deficit disorder. While on the drug sufferers experience fewer difficulties in concentration and maintaining attention. Use of the drug can provide a kind of "therapeutic trial," where the patient genuinely suffering from the disorder improves, while those mistakenly diagnosed develop only the side effects. Similar trials can be expected in the future that will resolve a most vexing issue: deciding when and under what circumstances people should be offered medications to solve life problems, and when they should be encouraged to take nothing and tough it out. I believe that additional understanding of brain chemistry will most likely reveal that our most intimate thoughts and feelings are the result of chemical processes, processes that can be modified by new drugs.

Traditionalists decry the use of drugs (I prefer the term *medica-*

tions, i.e., properly and legally prescribed substances, as opposed to illegal, unregulated "street" *drugs*) as a cop-out, an avoidance of the responsibility for self-determination. While I agree with the principle of self-determination, I have also witnessed the psychically debilitating effects of severe mental illness with its attendant despair and irresolution. As a result of his depression a depressed person is powerless to do anything to help himself. All the more valuable, therefore, will be a means of distinguishing seriously paralyzing depressions from mild and limited depressive episodes, perhaps no more than temporary "blue" periods. When observations and interviews fail to make such distinctions, a patient's response to medications can be a useful tool.

Our present concepts about personality, normal and otherwise, will eventually have to be revamped to include the chemical dimension, which until now has either been ignored or haphazardly manipulated by "recreational" drugs aimed at temporary modifications of mood and behavior. Self-description and description of others will include information relating to the neurotransmitter pathways that help define us. "Self-esteem," for instance, will be defined in terms of a genetic constitution toward high or low self-estimation. Such excursions into the psychophysiological are not new: we refer to some people as "adrenaline freaks," an imprecise but intuitive appreciation of the importance of that neurotransmitter in their lives. But rather than implying a grim determinism, such knowledge will enhance human freedom since each person will have the opportunity to alter important aspects of himself.

Some respond with reservations, or even fright, to the opportunity to exert some measure of control over the workings of their own brain. "Drugs should not alter one's basic personality, it's essentially who we are," is the most common expression of this view. But who is to decide what constitutes one's basic personality? Most people would have no problem with the dispensing of a drug capable of restoring the shattered personality of the Alzheimer's patient. Nor are there many objections to the use of antipsychotic drugs capable of doing away with hallucinations and delusions in a schizophrenic. It's the alteration of "normal" personalities that gives rise to controversy. But is it "normal" for a person to become so frightened at the prospect of speaking before a sales conference that he'll do almost anything to get out of it, thus jeopardizing his advancement and career? Medications already exist that can help such a person, and even more sophisticated ones are promised in the future.

Rather than illnesses, various difficulties or problems in living will be targeted. Thus advances in our understanding of the brain, a scientific endeavor, will have an impact on humanistic issues; for the first time we will have the means to change those parts of our personality into an ideal of our own choosing. But since such choices will inevitably reflect society's current ideas about the "good life" and society's value judgments, our newfound medication-induced freedom may not be as liberating as we anticipate. Workaholics, anorexics, and various seekers of one kind of "perfection" or another will have available to them the chemical means of working longer and harder, eating less, and achieving more through single-minded dedication to increasingly narrow tasks. Already controversies are breaking out regarding some students' use of medications for the concentration difficulties attending their attention deficit disorders. When they take their medicine prior to a test they can concentrate better and score higher. But is that fair to the others, some parents are asking. Is such medication the equivalent of steroid use in athletes?

The questions raised by the new brain-altering chemicals will also influence our ideas of right and wrong and how our judicial system decides such matters. Is violence the result, as some are claiming, of a shortage of serotonin in the frontal lobes? And if indeed the frontal lobes of a murderer are found to contain less serotonin than normal, does that mean he is not responsible for the murders he has committed? This is not just a rhetorical question. Three weeks from the time I am writing these words I will be testifying as an expert witness in a court hearing to determine whether a man who has been tried and convicted of the murder of eight prostitutes should be executed or spend the rest of his life in prison.

Sitting before me on my desk is the report of another expert called by the defense, who is suggesting just such a correlation between a frontal lobe deficiency of serotonin and the accused's powerlessness to avoid stalking and killing his victims. His testimony rests on some research in animals that suggests that serotonin plays a role in behavioral inhibition, and that a decrease in this neurotransmitter leads to an inability to adopt passive or waiting attitudes toward frustrations, or to inhibit aggressive actions in the face of threatened punishment (the frequently mentioned failure to "learn from experience").

In humans there is also evidence of serotonin's role in aggression and violence. Lower levels of serotonin's breakdown product (the chemical 5-HIAA or hydroxy indole acetic acid) appear in the spinal fluid of aggressive criminal offenders than in those with less aggressive incidents. Aggression against the self—suicide—also seems more common in people who have decreased levels of serotonin or 5-HIAA in their brain stem and cerebrospinal fluid. As a further indication of the role the lack of serotonin plays in violent behavior, consider that many of the medications useful for impulsive and aggressive disorders affect the serotonin system. And other disorders marked by problems with inhibiting certain impulses (kleptomania, pathological gambling, and self-injuring or self-mutilating behaviors) appear to be associated, at least on occasion, with lowered serotonin levels.

Based on correlations between lowered serotonin levels and some forms of violence, the opposing expert is testifying that the perpetrator, who is accused of carrying out a particularly gruesome and calculated series of murder mutilations (he dismembered several of his victims), suffers from a neurological disease. Yet several researchers reached the following conclusion about the serotonin-violence correlation:

"The serotonin hypothesis of impulsivity is therefore perhaps best conceived of as an initial research model rather than a definitive model. Neurobiological research on impulse control disorders is in its infancy. . . . The relative lack of work on the neurobiology of the impulse control disorders makes any conclusions about their mechanisms tentative."

In short, a suggestive but unproven research model is being offered by the defense as a preferable theory of behavior rather than the concept of personal responsibility that is the underpinning of our judicial system. (The convicted serial killer originally pleaded insanity, a legitimate impairment of personal responsibility, but that plea was rejected by the jury, who found him guilty, and the judge, who condemned him to death.) This is a heavy, and I would suggest, ultimately inappropriate burden for the neurosciences to assume. If such an argument is accepted, our concept of good and evil will have to be replaced by notions having to do with neurotransmitter imbalance— a situation, in short, that will doom our traditional ideas about personal accountability to the rubbish heap.

While knowledge about the brain can provide help and direction in understanding social problems like serial killers and widespread violence, its validity as a moral arbiter is highly debatable. Serotonin, along with the other neurotransmitters, is a complex system involving multiple receptor subtypes and complex interactions with a so far undetermined number of other neurotransmitter systems. A degree of humility is called for, the humility of the man or woman who is comfortable enough to say: "We have learned much but there is still much that we do not know. Therefore we will be cautious and not make claims that our present knowledge about the brain cannot support."

Over the next two decades other challenging and intriguing developments can be expected in the neurosciences. Perhaps the most promising is nerve cell transplantation. By surgically implanting brain parts in affected patients, formerly untreatable or unresponsive behavioral illnesses will be brought under control.

Many people cringe at the notion of brain surgery as a means of curing neurological disorders, recalling the spate of "psychosurgical" operations carried out in the 1950s and 60s. Such operations, often performed in the interests of ideology rather than scientific research, resulted in thousands of tragically impaired people. But transplantation surgery is an utterly different matter.

The most common transplant operation, already in use today on a limited basis, is aimed at helping victims of Parkinson's disease. Patients afflicted with this degenerative brain disease display a host of symptoms and signs resulting from a deficiency of the neurotransmitter dopamine. They move slowly and stiffly in a caricature of old age, even down to the characteristic tremor of their hands. Victims of Parkinson's seem out of touch with others since their faces, often compared to masks, display little emotion, and their voices, often barely audible, vary little in tone or timbre, no matter what the topic of conversation. In addition, the typical Parkinson's patient is bent over at the waist and walks with a shuffling, agonizingly slow gait.

With replacement of the deficient neurotransmitter dopamine, many of the signs of Parkinson's disease improve. In most cases this replacement consists of a daily dose of pills containing L-dopa, which upon entering the brain is transformed into dopamine. But for some Parkinson's patients, such medication doesn't work, and a neural transplant operation is their only hope.

Typical of such patients was Donald Wilson, who eventually became so incapacitated by his Parkinson's that he had to crawl on his hands and knees in order to navigate across his bedroom. Eventually the tremors and rigidity of his limbs grew so disabling that he spent the greater part of his waking hours in a wheelchair. In desperation Wilson offered to become the first American to have dopamine-producing brain tissue taken from an aborted fetus transplanted into his brain. After his operation Wilson was again able to walk and returned to his hobby of woodworking in his shop outside of Denver. Wilson's operation and others like it raise not only issues of technical difficulty, but ethical sensitivity as well. Many Americans equate abortion with murder, and even those who don't hold this view are still uncomfortable about using fetal tissues for transplantation.

A promising solution to this impasse may be forthcoming from recent developments in genetics. In the foreseeable future a person's skin cells may be able to be genetically modified so as to "turn on" the genes responsible for producing dopamine. This new approach is based on the fact that, as we have seen, with the exception of blood cells, every one of the body's trillions of cells carries the same genetic program.

Other promising approaches include the use of genetically altered cells to produce brain chemicals missing or deficient in brain diseases; the grafting of special virus-containing cells in the brain, which will be genetically engineered to produce the chemicals missing in a disease such as Alzheimer's; and the use of brain cells from other species. Already Brown University's Dr. Patrick Aebischer has come up with a clever way of introducing brain cells from one species into another by placing the cells in a special polymer material containing holes large enough to let brain chemicals out but small enough to block the entry of antibodies and thus prevent rejection.

"Neural transplantation in experimental animals serves as a useful tool with which to study brain function," says Fred H. Gage of the Department of Neurosciences at the University of California–San Diego. "Ultimately, such research may lead us to a clearer understanding of the changes that occur in the brain with normal aging, Alzheimer's disease, and dementia."

But neural transplantation is only a second-best approach to understanding and curing degenerative brain diseases. Top priority must be given to determining the actual causes of these diseases.

One recent branch of research in this area has investigated the alarming number of chemicals in our environment that, as it's becoming increasingly clear, are capable of producing brain injury. Moreover, many of these injurious effects often go unrecognized, because the symptoms are subtle and may not appear for months or even years. Brain injuries secondary to poisons in the environment may induce anxiety, confusion, psychosis, memory loss, convulsions, and even death. There are several reasons why the brain is particularly vulnerable to poisons. Unlike other cells in the body, nerve cells normally do not regenerate. Toxic damage to the brain is therefore usually permanent. Secondly, many neurotoxic substances cross easily into the brain. Since normal brain function depends on the maintenance of an exquisitely balanced mixture of chemicals, any entry of foreign chemicals has the potential to interfere seriously with normal function. Even minor changes in the structure or function of the nervous system can produce a kind of *Silent Spring* of the brain, which includes far-ranging aberrations in behavior. Early brain damage during fetal development may not make itself known until late in life, when the brain's capacity is compromised.

Manganese, an essential metal, is a prime example of a neurotoxin that produces a constellation of neurologic difficulties. Manganese workers inhale the ore dust in the mines, which then travels from the lungs to the brain where it accumulates within the basal ganglia. As a result some workers exhibit the slowness and tremors characteristic of Parkinson's disease. Others experience the onset of inappropriate and inexplicable bouts of laughing and weeping (an indicator of the subcortical origin of spontaneous expressions of emotion). But even in workers exposed to low levels of the element, psychological tests are often abnormal despite the absence of other symptoms. The workers are often unduly irritable, chronically fatigued, and complain of ringing in the ears and trembling of the hands.

In the section on neurotransmitters we mentioned another class of neurotoxins, inhibitors of the enzyme acetylcholinesterase, which breaks down the neurotransmitter acetylcholine. Many pesticides are designed to attack the nervous system of insects by altering the breakdown of acetylcholine. Not surprisingly, these agents also act on our own brains and nervous systems to produce symptoms like weakness, difficulty in breathing, visual disturbances, and, in some cases, explosive violence. With low rates of exposure the problems are more subtle: a prevailing sense of tension, disturbed sleep, restlessness, chronic anxiety, and nervousness when standing in lines.

"The implications of behavioral toxicology are profound," explains Bernard Weiss of the Department of Environmental Medicine at the University of Rochester School of Medicine and Dentistry. Weiss speaks of "silent toxicity," a term referring to illnesses that don't develop until many years after exposure and that cannot be detected without sophisticated psychological tests. "Another example might be the emergence of neurodegenerative diseases late in life, when the diminished reserve capacity of the brain is no longer sufficient to compensate for damage inflicted years earlier. We have little idea of the possible contribution of environmental poisons to these diseases, which begin long before they burst into clinical visibility," says Weiss.

Most worrying of all is the possibility that some of the degenerative brain diseases that are increasing in frequency (Parkinson's and Alzheimer's, to name only two) may result from so far unidentified toxins in our environment.

Even chemicals that we eat, both natural and synthetic, can exert devastating effects on the adult brain. Foods like the drought-resistant grain pea can induce a disease marked by gradual paralysis and eventual death. The active ingredient in the pea is thought to be an excitatory amino acid that, after ingestion, attacks certain parts of the brain. Such food-induced brain diseases are not limited to distant and exotic parts of the world. In 1987, in Canada, mussels contaminated with the excitatory neurotoxin domoic acid led to 129 illnesses and 2 deaths. Symptoms included memory loss, disorientation, and seizures.

A valuable spinoff of research on neurotoxins will be the identification of people with an decreased susceptibility to environmental toxins. Examples of this are known to all of us: the person who can smoke a pack or more of cigarettes per day over a long life span and yet never develop any of the tobacco-associated illnesses that kill hundreds of thousands of people per year who smoked more moderately. Toxins are not equal-opportunity destroyers. One person's bad habit is another person's death sentence.

Over the next decade neuroscientists will attempt to discover mechanisms of action of neurotoxins at the brain-cell level. If successful their efforts will confer a double benefit. Not only will neurotoxic effects be understood and combated, but the use of in-vitro methods (i.e., studies done outside the body) will cut down on the need for human and animal research. Neuroscientists will be looking for and, I predict, finding evidence that some neurologic and psychiatric diseases result from toxins in our everyday environment.

So far, appeals to clean up our external environment have gone largely unheeded, even when these appeals have been bolstered by indications of transgenetic effects that may harm our children and our grandchildren. Will these appeals be any more successful if we learn that toxins in our environment may, in fact, be destroying our minds today?

VI

At various times I have referred to the brain as the preeminent information processor. Indeed, the brain processes information at every level of its functioning. Traditionally and out of habit we have come to think of information as consisting of words, symbols, numbers, diagrams, and other products of our brain's reading and writing capacities. But this is much too narrow a definition; information is also contained in chemical formulas, electrical activity, and the coordinated actions of neuronal circuits. Let me illustrate this point by an example:

If you attend one of my public readings of this book my words, the elementary symbols of communication, travel as sound waves that impinge upon the tympanic membrane of your ears, where the message is converted into nerve impulses. From my end, this involves a conversion process whereby the symbolism imparted by words is converted into sound-wave frequencies created by the movements of my tongue and lips.

Upon arrival at the primary auditory reception area in the temporal lobe of your brain the message passes to the auditory association cortex and into the other association areas. (Recall the example earlier in the book of looking at an image from three inches away. As you step back and put the colors and forms into meaningful relationships, the information content of your perceptions is enormously enhanced. This is brought about by the recruitment of many brain areas connected via the association cortex.) The information contained in my words also travels into your limbic system, where the message takes on emotional value: You don't just hear words but react to them as well. PET scans reveal that many more areas of the brain are involved than was traditionally thought in an activity as seemingly straightforward as listening to an author read from his book (a neat refutation of the oft repeated canard that we only use one tenth of our brain).

If we drop down to the cellular level, the words you are hearing are probably already encoded in the form of networks of neurons. The symbolism of the words is present here as well, but in the form of neuronal firing patterns. With repetition, the patterns are strengthened and the information more firmly encoded, such as happens in the formation of habits which, essentially, are facilitated neuronal networks that have been repeated again and again.

Dropping down to the molecular level the symbolism of my spoken words is translated within your brain into the ebb and flow of neurotransmitters as they pass from a presynaptic neuron into the synapse and make the journey across to their receptors on the postsynapatic cell.

Words are thus translated into nerve impulses, into neuronal networks, and into the flow of neurotransmitters—these are the information transformations that occur at the three levels of the brain. But how does one interrelate the symbolism at these three levels? With this question we come up against the greatest and most intractable challenge of brain research. Although thoughts readily translate into words, no one so far has been able to understand how thoughts are transformed into the action of networks of neurons, perhaps several hundred million at a time, or into the blending of the action of fifty to a hundred neurotransmitters presently known (ignoring, for now, the existence of other as yet to be discovered chemical messengers). Is understanding the brain simply a matter of learning more about the three levels of brain functioning, applying it, and thus coming up with the necessary correlations? Or do we run up against an intractable obstacle here, a translation that will resist our best efforts?

Although I remain confident of our power to learn more and more about the brain I don't believe we will ever be able to make one-to-one correlations between the symbolism of thought, the symbolism of neuronal networks, and the actions of neurotransmitters.

Consider, for example, that the same symbols that convey our thoughts don't readily translate into single words: there are many ways of saying the same thing. Likewise, many different neuronal circuits can be enlisted to accomplish similar purposes. You may choose to walk across the room to turn on the television, or you may rely strictly on your brain's speech and language areas and ask someone else to do it for you. While the end result is the same, the neuronal circuitry involved differs enormously as does, it seems reasonable to expect, the blend of neurotransmitters involved. Moreover, even if such a correlation were made linking words to neuronal circuits to neurotransmitters, the meaningfulness and utility of such correlations would remain problematic. Would you be satisfied if you came to me for consultation about your loneliness and depression and I explained everything to you in terms of neurotransmitters? Of course not. You don't *experience* yourself in terms of chemistry but in thoughts, words, and feelings. These are not *things* but processes that exist only within our conscious awareness.

Though our inner states of awareness can be changed by chemicals—one has only to take a drink or have prescribed one of the newer antidepressants to experience this for oneself—such inner modifications can only be pursued a limited distance within the dynamic networks of the brain. To this extent the brain may turn out to be fathomable only to a certain degree, just as the physics of everyday reality, if pursued deeply enough, disappears into a blur of subatomic particles and fields of energy.

Finally there is the conundrum of the brain's understanding itself. We use our brains in order to understand the brain—a self-referential paradox that in moments of dispassionate appraisal creates doubts in the minds of even the most optimistic of neuroscientists.

In addition, our knowledge of the brain is limited by how we deal with three challenges: frame, scale, and category. Look at the drawing on page 128. The figures are set out seemingly at random. Yet if you look at the frames provided for these figures on page 128 you observe that the figures are not disordered, and that the order varies according to the frame imposed. In a similar way, our understanding of the brain varies according to whether we impose a neurochemical or an anatomical or a behavioral frame to highlight our observations. And just as the frames for the figures remain distinct and don't overlap one another, so, too, may the information we gain from, say, the neurochemical frame not be directly translatable to the anatomical or the behavioral. Each frame provides a unique way of understanding the brain; none is "better" or more complete than the other; they are different rather than qualitatively distinguishable.

The category challenge is related to the frame challenge. The

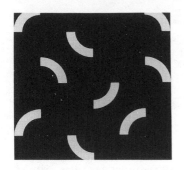

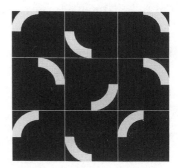

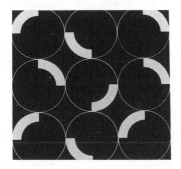

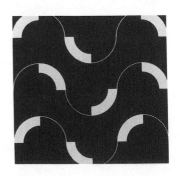

philosopher Gilbert Ryle explained it first, and the following can be considered an updated modification of his analogy. A young girl of eight or nine years of age is taken on a class trip to Washington, D.C., in order to see "how the government operates." Over the course of the day she visits the White House, Congress, and the Supreme Court. At the conclusion of her visit she confounds her hostess by inquiring, "But where is the government actually located?" Of course, there is no other response than to point out that "government" is a functional term employed in a totally different category of discourse than the components that constitute it. Mind and brain are often interchanged in this way, though no mind has ever been discerned in the absence of a brain, and indeed, the mind is best defined as the functional expression of the living brain.

Finally, our understanding must somehow come to grips with the scale problem. As you move your eyes along this sentence, the words are transformed into nerve signals that travel back along the optic nerve into several language and speech modules. Key neurons in these modules undergo changes in the permeability to ions, which generate the nerve signal, transforming it at the synapse into a chemical message conveyed by any number of neurotransmitters acting at receptors and their wide variety of subtypes. At this level the symbolism of words has been transformed into a symbolism of chemical affinity between neurotransmitter and receptor. Additional communication of symbolism is then conveyed by billions of nerve cells interacting together within networks. Thus the infinitely small, indeed the submicroscopic, combines with a near infinity of possible combinations that exceeds the capabilities of the most powerful of computers. While the brain can and has been studied at all of these levels, we often forget that our knowledge of the mechanisms of one of them, or even of all of them working together, does not really help us to grasp how these words are finally understood. To "understand" the brain we would have to somehow incorporate all of these scales into a unity while at the same time considering each of them simultaneously. An understanding of the brain must involve not only all three challenges of frame, category, and scale but also the paradox of self-reflection. At home I have a poster that displays a face reflected in what appears to be an infinity of mirrors. Beneath the figure is the caption: "Self-reference is the infinite in finite guise." Nowhere is self-reflection seen more clearly than in the brain, and consciousness lies at its basis. A PET scan of your brain taken this very moment would show activity in the visual and visual association areas corresponding to your reading of the sentences. It would also show activity in the frontal areas, where some degree of conscious processing is going on. If I call your attention to this frontal activity and accompany it with the suggestion that you concentrate deeply on some problem or other, you will witness a further development of the frontal activity, reflecting the enhanced conscious processing you are then carrying out. When we become conscious of our own mental activity the process is like the infinity of self-reflecting mirrors. There is no means of stepping back from this reality—leaving the frame, so to speak—since all aspects of mind require the activation of the brain. Each reflects the other with the greatest consciousness resulting from the most enhanced self-reflection.

But such reflections should not engender an attitude of nihilism. Recently neuroscientists have made great progress in advancing our understanding of the brain. Moreover they have established connections and correlations spanning the continuum from behavior to neuronal connections to chemical transmission and, finally, to a person's genetic constitution. An example of the new insights provided by brain science concerns an illness we all dread: Alzheimer's disease.

Until very recently dementia—popularly referred to as senility—was considered a normal part of aging. We know now that this is a mistaken notion. Artists like Picasso and scientists like Einstein illustrate the point that creativity and intellectual acumen can continue into a person's sixties or seventies, and beyond. In truth dementia is a disease, and like all diseases it has a cause. More than 60 percent of people with dementia suffer from Alzheimer's disease. As with many neurological diseases the diagnosis of Alzheimer's depends upon the demonstration at autopsy of characteristic microscopic changes in the brain.

The disease's discoverer, Alois Alzheimer, reported in 1907 on his observations of the brain of a middle-aged woman who died after a four-year history of progressive memory loss and a severe decline in her general mental functioning. Her brain was small and shriveled and had suffered a severe loss of neurons. While examining the cerebral cortex under a microscope, Alzheimer observed two distinct microscopic abnormalities. The first looked like tangles of barbed wire; in addition to these neurofibrillary tangles (NFT) the patient's brain contained smudgelike bodies that Alzheimer named senile plaques (SPs, also called neuritic plaques). In the intervening years these two abnormalities have become the official pathological markers of the disease that bears Alzheimer's name, and the density of the tangles and plaques has been found to correlate with the seriousness of the disease.

Sixty-seven years later neuroscientists made a discovery that put Alzheimer's observations into perspective. They found that the cerebral cortex and hippocampus of the brains of patients who died from Alzheimer's contained less than normal amounts of choline acetyltransferase (ChAT), the enzyme responsible for producing the neurotransmitter acetylcholine. The level of ChAT was far below that

found in normal aging people, and the degree of enzyme loss correlated directly with the severity of the dementia. Even more intriguing was the finding that both of these variables correlated with the
number of senile plaques in the hippocampus of the Alzheimer's
brain.

Acetylcholine plays an important role in memory, the mental
process that is most disturbed in Alzheimer's. If a normal college
volunteer is given a dose of the cholinergic antagonist scopolamine
she will suffer a striking temporary inability to form new memories.
This observation suggests a mechanism for memory loss in
Alzheimer's, which is now believed to result from the loss of acetyl-
choline-forming cells at the base of the brain toward the front, in the
so-called basal forebrain. While this theory accounted for the neurochemical aspect of the illness, it did nothing to clarify the meaning
of the senile plaques. That explanation would come from a most
unlikely source.

Children with Down's syndrome rapidly accumulate senile
plaques and neurofibrillary tangles. By age thirty-five their brains
resemble those of people with advanced Alzheimer's. The genetic
abnormality responsible for Down's consists of three copies of chromosome 21 rather than the normal two copies. Inherited forms of
Alzheimer's often can be traced by linkage studies to an abnormality
on that same chromosome. Chromosome 21 also contains a gene
encoding for a large protein, amyloid precursor protein, that is
necessary for normal brain development and neuron-to-neuron communication. Amyloid, it turns out, is an abnormal by-product resulting from the breakdown of amyloid precursor protein. Extra copies
of a gene on chromosome 21 are responsible for an accelerated and
enhanced breakdown of amyloid precursor protein, a resulting

increase in the production of amyloid, and an accompanying increase in the generation of a toxic by-product of amyloid that kills brain cells and produces Alzheimer's.

While this finding illuminates the nature of inherited Alzheimer's, it is of little help in explaining the much more common late-onset form of the disease, which occurs sporadically and is not inherited. The genetic abnormality here resides on a different chromosome (19) and is associated with an abnormality of a different protein known as apolipoprotein, which is associated with the transport of cholesterol and the normal development of the brain. Accumulation of an abnormal form of this protein is found in the plaques and neurofibrillary tangles found after death in the brains of patients with a late onset of Alzheimer's.

Thus two different chromosome abnormalities can produce identical disease states. This is one of the reasons most researchers have given up on the idea that such a complex disorder as Alzheimer's will ever be explainable on the basis of a single gene or a single neurotransmitter. As well as genetic factors, several environmental factors also play a role in the development of the disease. An advanced education, the use of nonsteroidal anti-inflammatory drugs (NSAIDs) like Advil, and smoking decrease the risk of contracting the disease. The better-educated person has more resources to stimulate his engagement and interest in the world around him—another example of the "use it or lose it" principle that underlies all brain functioning from the moment of our birth. The correlation with smoking is based on the fact that nicotine occupies its own subtype of acetylcholine receptor and acts as a trophic (stimulating) factor in generating an increase in the total number of acetylcholine receptors. Such a discovery immediately presents an ethical dilemma: a doctor can hardly suggest smoking as a preventative for Alzheimer's, since it is known to produce other perils such as lung cancer and emphysema. (So far the positive effects of NSAIDs remains unexplained.)

No one is certain at this point how the accumulation of amyloid leads to the destruction of neurons and the devastating mental regressions that characterize Alzheimer's. But the findings so far suggest an important principle: A continuum exists from the molecular to the behavioral. One can start with the genes and work outward toward the behavioral: the memory loss, disorientation, and other disabling features of Alzheimer's. Or one can begin at the other end of the continuum and work inward to inner domains of the nerve cell: experience influencing brain systems, which influence circuits, which influence synaptic relationships, which influence ion channels, which influence neurotransmitters, which influence second-messenger systems, which, finally, influence genes to change structure and function. Alzheimer's research, with its varied approach spanning the behavioral to the molecular, is a model for how brain research is likely to develop in the foreseeable future.

"Even in an illness that is genetically determined, environmental factors can play an important role in modifying the genetic vulnerability," said Joseph T. Coyle of the Department of Psychiatry at McLean Hospital in Boston. Why should this be surprising? While the brain depends for its functioning upon its genetic endowment, genes must express themselves within and be influenced by an environment. And while the brain operates via electricity and chemistry, it is also a product of the social and psychological world in which it finds itself. In short, all that we are and all that we can be cannot be considered separately from our brain. The philosopher Immanuel Kant, although he never spoke about the brain, expressed a similar belief when he suggested that we do not experience things as they are in themselves but only as filtered through the medium of the mind—we would now say the brain. This clearly implies a direct relationship between our brain's organization and operation and what we can learn about the world and about ourselves as part of that world.

Until recently few people other than neuroscientists knew much about the brain or felt any interest in learning more. Yet if, as the majority of neuroscientists now believe, we cannot consider our nature apart from the operation of our brain, which we employ in the exploration of such questions, what could be more worthy of our efforts, as we approach the third millennium, than to learn as much as we can about it?

Bibliography

Adelman, George, ed. *Encyclopedia of Neuroscience*. 2 vols. Cambridge, Mass: Birkhauser Boston, 1987.

Adelman, George, and Barry Smith, eds. *Neuroscience Year: Supplement 3 to the Encyclopedia of Neuroscience*. Cambridge, Mass: Birkhauser Boston, 1993.

Benson, D. Frank. *The Neurology of Thinking*. New York: Oxford University Press, 1994.

Black, Ira B. *Information in the Brain: A Molecular Perspective*. Cambridge, Mass: MIT Press, 1991.

Dressler, David, and Huntington Potter. *Discovering Enzymes*. New York: Scientific American Library, 1991.

Edelman, Gerald M. *Bright Air, Brilliant Fire: On the Matter of the Mind*. New York: Basic Books, 1992.

Finger, Stanley. *Origins of Neuroscience: A History of Explorations into Brain Function*. New York: Oxford University Press, 1994.

Gregory, Richard L., ed. *The Oxford Companion to the Mind*. New York: Oxford University Press, 1987.

Hyman, Steven E., and Eric J. Nestler. *The Molecular Foundations of Psychiatry*. Washington, DC: American Psychiatric Press, Inc, 1993.

Lyon, Jeff, and Peter Gorner. *Altered Fates: Gene Therapy and the Retooling of Human Life*. New York: W.W. Norton, 1995.

Posner, Michael I., and Marcus E. Raichle. *Images of Mind*. New York: Scientific American Library, 1994.

Restak, Richard M. *Receptors*. New York: Bantam, 1994.

INDEX

142   I N D E X